GULLIVER IN THE LAND OF GIANTS

Gulliver in the Land of Giants

A Critical Biography and the
Memoirs of the Celebrated Dwarf Joseph Boruwlaski

ANNA GRZEŚKOWIAK-KRWAWICZ

Warsaw University, Poland and the Polish Academy of Sciences

Translated by Daniel Sax

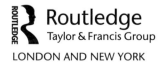

Routledge
Taylor & Francis Group

LONDON AND NEW YORK

First published 2012 by Ashgate Publishing

2 Park Square, Milton Park, Abingdon, Oxon OX14 4RN
711 Third Avenue, New York, NY 10017, USA

Routledge is an imprint of the Taylor & Francis Group, an informa business

First issued in paperback 2017

British Library Cataloguing in Publication Data
Grzeskowiak-Krwawicz, Anna.
  Gulliver in the land of giants : a critical biography and
  the memoirs of the celebrated dwarf Joseph Boruwlaski.
  1. Boruslawski, Jozef, 1739-1837. 2. Dwarfs--Poland--
  Biography. 3. Dwarfs--Great Britain--Biography. 4. People
  with disabilities and the performing arts--Europe--
  History--18th century. 5. People with disabilities and the
  performing arts--Europe--History--19th century.
  6. Enlightenment--Europe.
  I. Title II. Boruslawski, Jozef, 1739-1837.
  362.4'092-dc23

Library of Congress Cataloging-in-Publication Data
Grzeskowiak-Krwawicz, Anna.
  Gulliver in the land of giants : a critical biography and the memoirs of
the celebrated dwarf Joseph Boruwlaski / Anna Grzeskowiak-Krwawicz.
     p. cm.
  Includes bibliographical references and index.
  ISBN 978-1-4094-2033-0 (hardcover)
  1. Boruslawski, Jszef, 1739-1837. 2. Dwarfs--Poland--Biography.
  3. Favorites, Royal--Europe--Biography. 4. Boruslawski, Jszef,
  1739-1837--Travel--Europe. 5. Europe--Description and travel. 6.
  Enlightenment--Europe. 7. Europe--Intellectual life--18th century. 8.
  Salons--Europe--History--18th century. 9. Europe--Social life and
  customs--18th century. I. Title.

  CT9992.B67G79 2012
  943.8'025092--dc23
  [B]
                                                                    2011038473
  ISBN 978-1-4094-2033-0 (hbk)
  ISBN 978-1-138-10776-2 (pbk)

Contents

List of Plates

Acknowledgements

I would sincerely like to thank all the institutions that contributed to the development of this book and its final form. I am very grateful to the British Academy for a scholarship that enabled me to track down traces of Boruwłaski in England, to Durham University Library, the Chapter Library at Durham Cathedral, and the City Council of Durham, and to the Royal College of Surgeons of England for granting access to illustration material and consent for its publication. Apart from these institutions themselves I wish to thank their staff members for the interest they took in my work and all the kindness and assistance they showed me. I am indebted to Andrzej Suchcitz and Dr Krzysztof Stoliński for assistance and inspiration at the beginning of my research on Boruwłaski's story, and am grateful to Mr Alain Duperon for providing me with materials resolving the riddle of what subsequently happened to Boruwłaski's wife Isalina Barboutan and their daughter Georgiana Fanny.

This book could never have been written without the assistance, advice, and support of my husband Marek, who accompanies me on all my scholarly escapades with unswerving patience and a sense of humour.

Introduction

For years, tourists visiting the lobby of the town-hall building in the British town of Durham have been intrigued by a sculpture depicting an elderly gentleman of charming appearance, wearing elegant early 19th-century garb, bent over a guitar. One might think that this monument to Joseph Boruwłaski, depicting him dressed to attend an audience with King George IV in 1820, would not be all that extraordinary: Boruwłaski was, after all, one of Durham's most famous residents ever. He was mentioned at considerable length in Diderot's great *Encyclopédie* in the eighteenth century and later in the *Encyclopaedia Britannica* and many other lexicons, the press followed the events of his life as they unfolded, and when he died in 1837 reports were carried by nearly every English daily and then by newspapers on the continent. But Boruwłaski's fame was indeed of quite an unusual sort. The encyclopaedia entries about him cannot be found in the conventional way, since they are not listed under his own name, and the above sculpture might indeed not catch the eyes of passers-by at all if it were not for the fact that this smallish, 99-centimetre figure is in fact *life-sized*. It was Boruwłaski's extraordinary smallness that determined his life story and was the main source of his fame – he was the most famous dwarf in eighteenth- and early nineteenth-century Europe, and it was as such that he figured on the pages of various encyclopaedias and dictionaries (where he should be sought under the entries for *dwarf* in English, *nain* in French, or *zwerg* in German).

Some slight memory of Boruwłaski has survived to the present day both in Poland, where he was born, and England, where he spent more than half of his long, 98-year life. Certain mementos related to him are still preserved and displayed in Durham – his portrait, clothing, violin, and other personal effects. A few printed works on him have appeared over the years: a publication commemorating the 'little count' and the events of his life was printed in Durham to mark the 150th anniversary of his death, and a small brochure was also published in Ireland to commemorate his stay in Portarlington.[1] He was prominent enough to rate an entry in the nineteenth-century *Dictionary of National Biography*, and in the twenty-first century *Oxford Dictionary of National Biography*,[2] in 1902 his memoirs were republished in London by Henry Richard Heatley (who tried to draw together further supplementary information about Boruwłaski's life story)[3] and in 1937 he was listed in a Polish biographical dictionary.[4] One Polish author paid quite a bit of attention to him in her analysis of the place of dwarfs in old Polish society, although she based herself mainly on the first edition of his memoirs and fails to mention nearly the entire English period of his life.[5] Nowadays, quite a few references to Boruwłaski can be found on the Internet, where he continues to spark interest as a kind of freak of nature – and indeed, it was mainly such a role that has been ascribed to him in the collective consciousness. If Boruwłaski was and is remembered, it is as he was depicted in the *Encyclopédie* and how he was perceived in the eighteenth century, as a misfit noteworthy for his oddity. Confirmation of this can be found in the fact that a fragment devoted to him appeared in a recent book discussing 'mutants.'[6]

---

[1] T. Heron, *The Little Count Joseph Boruwlaski*, City of Durham, 1986; J.S. Powell, *Joseph Boruwlaski his Visit to Portarlington 1795*, York (no date of publication) – this is essentially a reproduction of a small fragment of Boruwłaski's memoirs describing his stay in Portarlington, supplemented by certain details uncovered by the publisher.

[2] Margot Johnson, 'Boruwlaski, Joseph, styled Count Boruwlaski (1739–1837)', *Oxford Dictionary of National Biography*, online edn, Oxford University Press, Sept 2004.

[3] *The Life and Love Letters of a Dwarf*, ed. H.R. Heatley, London, 1902. This publisher gathered the most supplementary information about Boruwłaski's life.

[4] S. Wasylewski, *Józef Boruwłaski*. In: *Polski Słownik Biograficzny*, vol. 2, Kraków, 1937, p. 356. This biographical entry consists almost exclusively of a quite haphazard summary of the memoirs. Wasylewski also devoted a popular essay '*Dama z karzełkiem*' to Boruwłaski in his book *Romans prababki*, Lwów, 1920.

[5] B. Fabiani, *Niziołki, łokietki, karlikowie*, Warsaw, 1980.

[6] A.M. Leroi, *Mutants: on the form, varieties and errors of the human body*, London, Harper Collins, 2003, pp. 170–177; This is also the standpoint from which Boruwłaski's life story is analysed by Barbara Benedict, the author of a notable article on him (B. Benedict, 'Displaying Difference: Curious Count Boruwlaski and the Staging of Class Identity', *Eighteenth-Century Life*, vol. 30, no. 3, summer 2006, pp. 78–106), which unfortunately does not take account of the original Polish version of the present biographical essay, published two years previously (A. Grześkowiak-Krwawicz, *Zabaweczka: Józef Boruwłaski – fenomen natury – szlachcic – pamiętnikarz*, Gdańsk, Słowo/obraz-terytoria, 2004).

And yet it seems that an attempt deserves to be made to consider Boruwłaski's life and the description of it he left behind in his memoirs not only more thoroughly and penetratingly, but also from somewhat of a different perspective. To look upon him not just as a member of a separate society of Lilliputians – as a curious natural phenomenon – but as a sensitive and intelligent man in his own right, in a certain sense imprisoned within his own body, just as much by nature as by the role imposed upon him by 'society at large,' so to speak. This was a role that to some extent he was forced to accept and which indeed brought him certain benefits, but which he spent his entire life rebelling against, going to great lengths to try to liberate himself from. Perhaps that is why in the last edition of his memoirs he likened himself to Gulliver exploring the world of giants; this was not just a witty literary reference but also a kind of role-reversal: he was no longer the one that differed from the norm; rather it was the whole world surrounding him that was abnormal. This is an ingenious perspective that merits closer investigation: looking at the world of the latter eighteenth and early nineteenth century through Boruwłaski's eyes is sure to yield a picture that is fresh and captivating, and at the same time astonishingly different from what we know about the cultural elite of the Enlightenment era.

Chapter 1

Dwarf of the Salons

At first glance, the fact that Joseph Boruwłaski left behind a sizeable set of published memoirs (the first version of which is included in the present volume) might seem to make the historian's task of retracing his life and fortunes relatively easy. He even revised and expanded his written recollections several times to include subsequent years. Nonetheless, for the careful and cautious historian the job in fact proves to be much harder, despite this relatively plentiful material. Boruwłaski's autobiographical writings need to be taken with a considerable grain of salt, so to speak, especially in this later period – when it seems the author wished to portray his life according to a certain image he had always held in his imagination, omitting many events, distorting others, and quite simply fabricating still others. He moreover sometimes dates events inaccurately, or more often (wanting to additionally cover up his real tracks?) he cautiously avoids giving any dating whatsoever. Admittedly, the earlier edition of the memoirs does represent a more credible historical source (although as we will discuss below, it too represents a kind of literary creation, and quite a successful one at that). When this first portion was initially published, nearly all the individuals involved in the depicted events were still alive and the memoirs were even expressly addressed to some of them, hence the stories are naturally retold more scrupulously and accurately. But this portion unfortunately goes no further than 1788–1790.

The present work grew largely out of research work contrasting the various versions of Boruwłaski's memoirs to one another with a critical eye and confronting them against other historical sources, for example, accounts left behind by individuals who knew Boruwłaski, press reports, and preserved personal correspondence, in order to retrace and recount the course of his life as accurately as possible.

In this vein, we should start by dealing with the fundamental issue of our subject's name itself and clearing up some potential misunderstandings here. Firstly, this book uses the English first name 'Joseph,' by which he was known in later years, although the reader should bear in mind that his true first name was in fact the Polish 'Józef.' Secondly, the issue of his surname has proven considerably more problematic over the years. Certain readers may wonder whether it really should be 'Boru*wła*ski' (roughly pronounced *bor-oo-VWAH-ski*, as the Polish crossed-L letter is pronounced like an English 'w'), as used in this book, or perhaps the more naturally Slavic-sounding configuration 'Boru*sław*ski' – especially since the latter form is indeed frequently found in writings about him in nineteenth- and twentieth-century Poland? Although the first version does fall somewhat awkwardly even upon the Polish ear, we can nevertheless confirm that it is without any doubt the true and correct form: Boruwłaski used precisely this spelling in signing not only his own memoirs but also his personal letters, including ones addressed to Poles, and moreover in his lifetime he was widely known as 'Boruwłaski' throughout Europe. In a certain sense, further confirmation that this more awkward rendering is the correct one can be found in the broad range of other distortions and misspellings that have appeared over the years – ranging from 'Borwslasky' in Count de Tressan's writings to the entry in Diderot's *Encyclopédie* dealing with 'Borwilasky.' Here credit is due to the British for distorting the name relatively infrequently, presumably because they were in closest contact with both the man and his name in later years, and were better aware of the correct spelling from his published memoirs themselves and from newspaper reports. But then again, who knows whether certain positive connotations might have also played a certain part here? At least to the Scots, his name is reported to have conjured up an association with 'barrel-o-whisky,' and this is allegedly how it was pronounced during Boruwłaski's stay in Edinburgh in 1788.

Although Boruwłaski was frequently described as bearing the title 'count,' he in fact bore no aristocratic peerage and made no such claim. Rather, his use of the term 'count' in press announcements or in the final edition of his memoirs, it seems, served more to underscore his noble origins and to drive that point home to his title-accustomed Western readers. In reality Boruwłaski was born in 1739 into a family of petty nobility that struggled to make ends meet, and he never made any secret of that fact. While mention was sometimes made of a former family fortune his father had once lost, either in the service of Polish King Stanisław Leszczyński or under other unspecified circumstances,[1] the only certainty is that his was a poor family, especially after his father's death when Joseph was just 9 years old. Their poverty was all the more tragic in that no less than three of the six children were of Lilliputian size – Joseph's elder brother exceeded him only slightly in height, and their sister, three years Joseph's younger, was even smaller than both her brothers at just 66 cm. Count de Tressan accused Boruwłaski's parents of having 'looked upon the two elder brothers like unfortunate whims of nature and left them without education,'[2] but this is an unfair assertion, as Boruwłaski's memoirs do not indicate he received any less care than his other siblings. The French count seems not to have fully realised what opportunities and needs a poor noble family in Poland's Pokucie province actually had to educate their children, whatever their height. On the other hand, there is no doubt that the future of these three little ones must have been an especially serious concern for their parents – their height shut them off even from the few routes to success that remained open for their normal-sized brothers: the clergy, military service, and favourable marriage. Nevertheless, there was one more possibility for social advancement, quite widespread in those times: service to a powerful lord, or at least to a wealthy gentleman. In this latter case an unusual physique could actually prove to be an asset, helping pique the interest of a potential benefactor or benefactress – the kind of person Helena Stadnicka, the later Countess Tarnowska, would indeed become for the young Joseph. Importantly, as Joseph stressed in his own memoirs and as is confirmed by all contemporary sources, the whole Boruwłaski trio were not just of small size but also of very attractive appearance and proportionally built, without any of the deformations or disabilities commonly found in dwarfs. It is no surprise, therefore, that all three ultimately found themselves sponsors – just as Joseph

---

[1]   *Gazeteer*, 19 Oct 1786; in the fourth and final edition of his memoirs the author writes about the loss of some estate on the Dnieper River – *Memoirs of Count Boruwlaski: containing a sketch of his travels, with an account at the different courts of Europe written by himself*, corrected by Mr Burdon, Durham: F. Humble, 1820, p. 15 (cited hereinafter as 'Memoirs IV').

[2]   L.E. de Tressan, *Mémoire envoyé à l'Académie Royale des Sciences par M. le Comte*, Paris, 1760. This quotation and others which follow are drawn from the translation of *Mémoire* included in this volume.

found sponsorship with Madame Helena Stadnicka, so too his brother found protection under the Castellane Ustrzycka of Inowłódz and the sister under the Castellane Katarzyna Kossakowska, a famous *hic mulier* known for her biting tongue. The Boruwłaski trio's small stature was undoubtedly the main motivation for the sponsorship of these noble ladies, who presumably wished to retain them as elegant playthings. However, their curious appearance did not in fact have to end up determining their entire career or the role they played throughout their whole lives: with time Joseph's elder brother, if we believe his memoirs, became a steward for Madame Ustrzycka, therefore enjoying what might otherwise be a successful career for a normal nobleman of modest means. Their sister, in turn, ended up in a role that was typical for people of her height for centuries, becoming Kossakowska's pet dwarf, but the position she eventually came to hold within the Castellane's retinue did not differ much from that of an ordinary lady-in-waiting – again, this was a role played by many poor noblewomen.

But it was Joseph whose life would prove to be the most colourful, and at the same time the most closely linked to his physical appearance. His rightful place in life was essentially already shown to him by Stadnicka – when she dubbed him 'Joujou,' or little toy. This nickname, appropriate for the child he then still was, and the role that went hand-in-hand with it would accompany him into his adult life as well. As one Polish scholar wrote in a short but brilliant analysis of the lives of similar dwarfs in the eighteenth century: 'Whether he liked it or not, the function of such a dwarf was to entertain the assembled company; that was what was expected of him. If he played that role well he would be rewarded and celebrated, if not, or if he did not wish to play such a role, he would fade into oblivion.'[3] Boruwłaski's chief task at this stage was to appeal as much as possible to the his masters, and this was something he realised quite quickly. 'I considered it as my duty to double my efforts, that I might render myself agreeable to the husband of my benefactress' – this is how he described his situation after Stadnicka's marriage to Jan Tarnowski. However, his great career as a 'dwarf of the salons,' as a source of court entertainment who amused the greatest monarchs of his era, truly got its start once the Countess Anna Humiecka, one of the wealthiest and most influential Polish ladies of her day,

---

3   J. Ryba, *Uwodzicielskie oblicza Oświecenia*, Katowice, 1994, p. 9.

took Boruwłaski under her wing at the age of 15 (or perhaps somewhat older, as the author's dating is somewhat haphazard here).

It was with Humiecka that he embarked on his first trip, on a grand tour around Europe, beginning in late 1758 or early 1759 with a visit paid to Maria Theresa's court in Vienna. After half a year there Humiecka set out with Boruwłaski for Munich, where they were warmly greeted by Elector Maximilian Joseph and his wife Maria Anna, the daughter of Polish King Augustus III. At the end of the same year they were hosted by the deposed Polish King Stanisław Leszczyński at his court in Lunéville. From there, in early 1760, they travelled to Paris where they spent more than a year, frequently visiting Maria Leszczyńska at Versailles and socialising with the best Parisian society. In spring of 1761 they set out on a return journey through the Netherlands, visiting the court in Lunéville again in August, and arriving, via Germany, back in Poland in autumn of the same year. We can say that Boruwłaski was fortunate that his protectress was such a *grande dame* of the age, able to introduce him into the royal courts and the world of salons. Or instead of using the phrase 'introduce him' perhaps we should state more precisely that she put him on display there – we should have no doubt (as Boruwłaski himself had no doubt) that his new protectress, although very caring, treated him as a plaything, like a rococo trinket to be shown off among high society. That is evident in the various accoutrements specifically used to enhance his peculiarity: he would get dressed up in showy costumes, frequently copies of military uniforms, such as one he called his 'big-baton colonel' uniform. The salon room of Humiecka's residence in Warsaw even contained something that amounted to a doll-house for her Joujou, which had a 'a small sofa, little tables, a small billiard set, and other games and toys.'[4] Such a living plaything was of even greater value if it had 'agreeable talents,' as Boruwłaski himself dubbed them. Thus Humiecka took great pains to ensure the education of her Joujou – he was taught to dance in Vienna by none other than Maria Theresa's own ballet-master Casparo Angiolini, and instructed to play the guitar in Paris by Pierre Gavinies, one of the most famous virtuosos of the day. He was then well prepared to dance the polonaise before Maria Theresa or to perform a Cossack dance on the table before the French princesses Victoire

---

4   K.T.H. [Klementyna z Tańskich Hoffmanowa], Józef Borusławski, *Przyjaciel Ludu*, vol. 5, Leszno, 1838, no. 12 / 22 Sept. 1838, p. 95 ff.

and Adélaïde in the court of their grandfather, Stanisław Leszczyński,[5] in every case to his audience's rapture. In fact he proved to be quite an able musician and when called to appear in public he would embellish his performances by playing the guitar and violin, sometimes even performing his own compositions. We must concede that the boy was also given certain general foundations of an education – Count de Tressan, describing him when he was 20 years old in 1759, wrote that he knew basic arithmetic, the dogmas of Catholic religion, passable German, and quite good French.

The latter fact was particularly important, as knowledge of French was in those times essential for entering the salons and participating in social discussion. The eighteenth century was an age of conversation – light and witty, captivating and charismatic, replete with paradoxes and adroit compliments, nimbly skipping from one topic to another, offering skilful speakers a chance to demonstrate their wit, the famous French *esprit*. It is telling how frequently the depiction in Boruwłaski's memoirs of his voyage with Humiecka keeps mentioning such conversation: Maria Theresa 'seemed much pleased with my reply,'[6] Stanisław Leszczyński 'asked several questions to which I gave satisfactory answers, seemed pleased with my replies,' Kaunitz was 'pretending that my conversations both amused and interested him,' and Maria Leszczyńska 'after having asked me many questions concerning the King her father, Bébé, and Poland, and our travels, she seemed pleased with my answers.' Considering his young age, we might entertain certain doubts about his real ability to make all the clever and flattering ripostes he describes in his memoirs, and about his claims to have enthralled Maria Theresa with them already at the very outset of his first journey. Nevertheless, this does not appear to be just empty boasting – the truth of his words seems to be borne out by the fact that he was still remembered in Vienna as much as 20 years later, as well as by the widespread fame he began to enjoy even before the end of his first voyage with Humiecka. Boruwłaski himself would later maintain it was his stay in Paris that ultimately perfected his refinement and rendered his

---

[5]   This latter episode occurred in August 1761 and was described by Fillion de Chagrineau in his account of princesses Victoire and Adélaïde's stay at their grandfather's court; cf. S. Gaber, *L'entourage polonais du roi Stanislas Leszczyński à Lunéville*, Nancy, 1972, p. 150.

[6]   This quotation and others which follow are drawn from the first edition of the memoirs, included in this volume.

conversation skills graceful and unaffected, but previously to that, during his visit to Stanisław Leszczyński's court, Count de Tressan had already described his talents in this field, writing that he 'participates in the most gracious manner in the subtle and witty exchange of views.' His talents in this regard are also confirmed by continued signs throughout his life of a well-developed sense of humour and ability to pay elegant compliments. He certainly knew how to use those abilities to curry favour with the high and mighty of the world when he had the chance, but as befits a true man-of-the-world he could also use them just to be gallant, with no self-seeking objective at all. For instance, when admiring a cascade in Killarney many years later while holding the helpful hand of a certain Irishman, he responded to the cries of the latter's wife – 'Take care, that that little gentleman does not fall' – by turning round and, after beholding a beautiful and lovely lady, responding: 'Madam, I fall already.'[7] He knew how to embody the very essence of courtly graciousness, albeit laced with just a touch of the risqué – many such ripostes can be found in Boruwłaski's memoirs and in others' reminiscences of him.

Essentially from the very moment he made his début at Maria Theresa's court, Boruwłaski shone in this role of a 'dwarf of the salons' (or perhaps 'rococo dwarf'), able to amuse every audience not only with his physical appearance but also with gracious conversation, clever compliments, and witty replies. We might say that he managed to get into the salons as a kind of freak-show, yet once there he earned himself admiration as a well-refined gentleman. He certainly knew how to win the hearts of rulers and their entourages. Austria's Maria Theresa, Stanisław Leszczyński and his daughter Maria the Queen of France, the Dutch Stadtholder, Polish King Stanisław Augustus, English Kings George III and IV – these are just some of his royal acquaintances, an impressive list many an aristocrat of the day could only have envied. However, it was not their opinion, but that of high society at large that ensured his popularity. In a certain sense he ideally fit the demands of his time, when it was no longer royal courts but rather the broader *beau monde* that set the standards of social values, when it was the acceptance of the high-society salons that was the ticket to fame.

The stance that the people of the age – or rather the elite of the age – took towards Boruwłaski is worthy of some deeper analysis, because it brings into

---

[7] *Memoirs* IV, p. 253.

excellent relief certain hallmarks of the prevailing customs as well as certain contradictions of the times. The interest shown in him, sometimes turning into outright fascination, was essentially paradoxical in that it ran counter to the professed aesthetic ideals of the Enlightenment. This was, after all, an epoch that rejected the Baroque age's unfettered imagination and vapid curiosity in anything different, strange, or monstrous. As Jean de la Bruyère wrote in his *Caractères*, 'The mania for collecting is a fondness not for what is good or beautiful but for what is rare and unique, for what one has and others have not. It is not a liking for what is perfect but for what is sought after, what is in vogue.'[8] This definition accommodates Boruwłaski's popularity very well – not to speak of truly baroque ideas like the Lilliputian feast once organised in Paris in his honour by the Farmer General Bouret, or his being served up to guests at table inside an 'urn' (a tureen or soup-dish) by Michal Kazimierz Ogiński. The latter act is largely reminiscent of another incident that occurred a century earlier at the behest of the Duke of Buckingham, who had his own dwarf Jeffrey Hudson served to table inside a pie. Despite what was widely proclaimed about the predominance of refinement and good taste, the people of the eighteenth century, whether they hailed from the elite or from the lower classes, still had just as much of an interest as their fathers and forefathers from previous centuries had had in all sorts of disabilities, deformities, physical defects, and anything that diverged from the norm. It suffices to glance at the press from those days to see how many advertisements there were announcing opportunities to come gaze at midgets, giants, bearded women, extremely obese or thin individuals, and so on. But while the plebs could still take a simple, genuine, and uninhibited interest in such matters, the elite now required some sort of exoneration. Boruwłaski, with his charm and intelligence, thus fit the bill ideally. There was nothing monstrous or grotesque about him; indeed his delicate build was a point of admiration. In 1760, the publisher of an English monthly wrote: 'He is well proportioned and has nothing shocking about him.'[9] Years later another writer would go a step further and state: 'His person and mind are complete models of elegance and refinement.'[10] He was different enough from normal to spark interest, yet at the

---

8　J. de la Bruyere, *Les Caractères*, Paris, 1951, p. 406. English version taken from http://www.ourcivilisation.com/smartboard/shop/bruyere/

9　*London Magazine*, April 1760, p. 130.

10　*Morning Herald*, 6 May 1786.

same time he fit excellently into the world where he functioned. Of course, by this we mean he fit into a certain specific place and into a certain specific role in this world.

To understand precisely what place and role these were, we must go back to Boruwłaski's stay in Lunéville in 1759 and to Count de Tressan's account of him (included in the present volume). This account is noteworthy as the earliest and most extensive source on Boruwłaski, which moreover served as the basis for many later publications: a summary of it appeared in the *Encyclopédie*, it was reprinted in the annals of the French Academy, cited in the press, and continued to be referenced by nineteenth-century writers.[11] More importantly, it illustrates very well how Boruwłaski was viewed by representatives of the social and intellectual elite of his day: de Tressan was not just a count and marshal in Leszczyński's court, but also a member of the French Academy, to which his report was addressed. The place ascribed to Boruwłaski is already signalled by his very first words: 'The Polish nobleman Mr Borwslasky [!] came to Luneville in the retinue of Countess Humiecka. [...] This young man may be considered the most curious being that nature has created; once one has come to know him, the Polish king's dwarf Bébé no longer has anything surprising about him.' Boruwłaski was therefore interesting as an even greater curiosity than Bébé; he fell into a certain group of anomalies, marvels of nature, and the virtues of his appearance or intellect would be noticed only in juxtaposition to another representative of the same group. Boruwłaski's own somewhat later statement about Maria Leszczyńska that 'she, till then, deemed the individuals of my species as ill-favoured by nature, as much in mind and intellectual faculties as in body, but that I had undeceived her in a very advantageous and pleasing manner' shows that he realised very well what kind of place had been ascribed to him. His memoirs often make quite bitter mention of 'individuals of my species,' or even 'our species,' endowed with certain traits. De Tressan even believed that unlike Nicolas Ferry (Bébé's real name), Boruwłaski was an ideal representative of his 'species.' The count admired the physical and intellectual differences between them, but in a certain sense these two dwarfs represented two different epochs and two different social roles. Ferry bore all the traits of a baroque court dwarf,

---

[11]   For example, E.J. Wood in *Giants and Dwarfs*, London, 1868, p. 335, gives a translation of broad fragments of de Tressan's report.

whose intellect was irrelevant because his physical defect was all that mattered. In that case, the fact he was not just of small size but also had a quite distinctly misshapen body essentially lent him added value. Every inch of Boruwłaski, on the other hand, embodied good taste and refinement. If he was a plaything, it was a perfect one. We can say that Count de Tressan admired him not because he was a dwarf, but specifically because of *what kind of dwarf* he was. The count admitted that Bébé was for him a source of disgust and instilled the kind of latent fear 'usually prompted by the degradation of our existence, while the young Pole, in contrast, instils pleasure with his appearance and intellect, he arouses interest in his feelings, and finally evokes just tenderness and a desire to soothe all pain and indignity such as his fate may entail.' Besides, it would be wrong to state that the count considered Boruwłaski just a plaything. De Tressan's attitude towards him was perhaps best voiced by the editor of an English newspaper, who, having cited fragments of the count's report, asserted that Boruwłaski would be an equally intriguing point of interest for a philosopher, for a 'man of taste,' as well as for ... an anatomist.[12] De Tressan did indeed look at Joujou with the delighted eye of the rococo man-of-the-salons, but at the same time, in keeping with the spirit of the Enlightenment, he tried to analyse and pin down the phenomenon that Boruwłaski represented. This distinctive mixture of perspectives is visible in his report, where he describes both Joseph's outward appearance and his knowledge, extols his physical as well as intellectual capabilities, and also writes about what he ate, how he slept, how he danced, and what his personality was like. On the one hand he speaks of Boruwłaski with respect as a young Polish nobleman, admires his refinement, and shows sincere sympathy for him, while on the other hand he does not hesitate to inquire about 'individuals who served him' and whether he was 'of full male virility' or to relish telling misleading tales about Boruwłaski and his siblings' deformities at the moment of their birth. The latter element, like the detailed description of Joseph's family, is de Tressan writing as an anatomist, attempting to explain the causes for an observed anomaly. Boruwłaski is here a 'case,' an interesting 'specimen' he recommends to his Academy colleagues for study. The philosopher in de Tressan, in turn, speaks up when the author admires how generously nature endowed its tiny creation, 'it even seems that she wanted to compensate him for his extremely

---

[12]   *Gazeteer*, 19 Oct. 1786.

small height with charms embellishing his entire personality, including ones we are continually discovering in his intellect.' We can say that while de Tressan looks upon Bébé as a freak of nature, Boruwłaski is for him more like a natural phenomenon. And not just for him; the same motif appears in other descriptions of Boruwłaski throughout his life, something he himself skilfully emphasised – the second edition of his memoirs was published with the English motto 'Mysterious nature who thy works shall scan / Behold a child in size in sense a man?' and various press announcements contained statements about how nature's creator could be admired even in his very smallest creations.

Essentially, in Count de Tressan's account we find to some degree an illustration of all three of Boruwłaski's roles: as an ornament of the salons, as an unusual 'case' of natural history, and lastly as a miracle of nature. We also find the earliest confirmation of his intelligence and cheerful character, attested by a friendly but objective witness.

It was presumably this brochure, which appeared in late 1759 or early 1760, that contributed to Boruwłaski's great popularity during his stay in Paris, especially because it was not just read by the scholarly academicians of its intended audience. It quickly reached all of high society, in the original or in reprints. Boruwłaski suddenly became fashionable and his fame even preceded him to the French capital, immediately generating great interest. Even before his arrival, the press (not just the French press) announced: 'A Polish lady is impatiently expected at Paris, who is bringing with her a Polish gentleman, who is two-and-twenty years old, and but sixteen inches high. He is every way well proportioned, and his understanding is well cultivated.'[13] In fact the author of this report somewhat overstated the point – Boruwłaski was at that time 28 inches tall. Still, he was shorter than Bébé, a fact he proudly stressed. Fashion was a hugely powerful force in eighteenth-century society, or at least among its upper crust; to be fashionable meant to be talked about, to have one's sayings repeated and one's company sought. In a word, to be fashionable meant to be at the very centre of high-society interest, and this was what Boruwłaski experienced. He writes, not without pride, that upon his return to Paris 'the curiosity I excited drew many visitors to my protectress [...] for in less than a week every person of high rank at court, and every person of fashion in town, waited upon her. I

---

[13] *Gazeteer*, 31 Dec. 1759.

cannot help expressing how infinitely I was flattered by this warm enthusiasm, and by the numberless civilities with which I was honoured.' In fact, it seems that this situation was not entirely pleasing to Humiecka, who in a way herself ended up overshadowed by the 'little wonder' she had wanted to show off in the salons of Europe. The announcement cited above already leaves little doubt about who was actually being impatiently awaited in Paris and being talked about there, and this reversal of roles is illustrated even better by a statement written by Madame Geoffrin, who while praising Boruwłaski in a letter to King Stanisław Augustus described his sponsor as the 'lady with the dwarf' (*'la dame au nain'*), clearly not even recalling her name.[14] Humiecka's dissatisfaction was evidenced by the harshness of her reaction to the quite impertinent behaviour of the Duchess of Modena – when inviting Humiecka to visit her she insisted that she should bring Joujou, or essentially ordered her to bring him along. Boruwłaski gives the best description of his own situation (although this is in reference to later events): 'I became as fashionable as a new dress just arrived for the ladies.'[15] Many years later, he would describe his successes in Paris in the final edition of his memoirs as if he had been there on his own, interacting with the best society as he himself saw fit, frequenting the intellectual salons and allegedly even meeting and astounding Voltaire himself while visiting Madame Geoffrin. However, this was just the commonplace projection of dreams onto the past. We can be certain he visited Geoffrin's salon just as he had gone everywhere, namely brought there by Humiecka to be exhibited and shown off. We can say that he was very much in vogue precisely like a fashionable dress, becoming the favourite plaything of high society for just one season. That is how he presented these experiences in the earlier edition of his memoirs.

It is hard to say how the 20-year-old boy he then was reacted to such success, but from the standpoint of his adult years one can sense he had certain mixed feelings. While he does proudly cite favourable opinions about himself, praise the impressions he made on successive individuals he met, and list the courtesies shown to him by representatives of the highest social circles, it does seem that he treated certain events as humiliating. This we can gauge in terms of what he

---

[14]   Marie Thérèse Geoffrin to Stanisław Augustus, 17 March 1771, in *Correspondance inédite du roi Stanislas Auguste Poniatowski et de Mme Geoffrin (1764–1777)*, ed. Ch. de Mouy, Paris, 1875, p. 398.

[15]   *Memoirs* IV, p. 315.

omits (later editions of his memoirs no longer mention the Cossack dance he performed on the table in Lunéville, or his being carried in Ogiński's urn, or the fight in which Bébé tried to throw him into the fireplace), although from time to time he does also point out his humiliations outright. The most appalling scene recounts a conversation held in Boruwłaski's presence about dwarfs' sexual capabilities and about the notion of mating him with his own sister as a test: 'from which I thought I had to conclude, not only that they believed themselves entitled to dispose of me without my advice, but even looked upon me as a being merely physical, without morality, on whom they might try experiments of every kind.' These are the most bitter words to be found anywhere in the memoirs. We can judge how strong an impression must have been evoked by 'the sort of contempt apparently implied in this project of uniting me with my sister,' by the fact that Boruwłaski expressed it a quarter-century afterwards, in memoirs that were addressed to the rich and powerful of his day and which essentially constituted more an apology than a criticism of their behaviour.

On the other hand, Boruwłaski's descriptions of his youth do not reveal much about his own emotions, offering instead more of an outsider's perspective on events, especially his dazzling career in the courts and salons. That perspective changes only once he begins to recount his experiences related to his return to Poland. Based on the memoirs we essentially can say very little about a nearly 20-year period (1761–1780), part of which he spent at Anna Humiecka's estate in Podole (which he does not mention at all), but a majority of which he spent with her in Warsaw. This was likely due to several factors. Although these were very turbulent times in Poland's history – including the Confederacy of Bar insurrection, a Russian intervention, and ultimately the first partition of Poland – they were nevertheless relatively calm years in Boruwłaski's life. As he writes in the final edition of his memoirs: 'In this state of tranquillity my days glided away, and I thought that no kind of vexation could disturb so happy a life.'[16] These times were also simply not as full of exciting events like visits to royal courts or galas thrown in his honour. Although it is undoubtedly true, as the writer notes, that his return to Poland 'made much noise' due to the fame he had gained during his travels, things here were similar to how they had been elsewhere and this interest was quite fleeting. Moreover, from his status as

---

[16]   Ibidem, p. 46.

the favourite marvel of the world's greatest salons, Boruwłaski now reverted
in a certain sense to his previous role. Regardless of the rapture he may have
instilled, he was still just Countess Humiecka's dwarf. In Warsaw the Countess
did not have to face any affronts similar to those in Paris, being an influential
lady well connected to Poland's most powerful families. King John III Sobieski
had been one of her ancestors on the distaff side and her brothers were active in
the current courtly circle: Kazimierz Rzewuski, famous for his good looks and
his duels, and Franciszek Rzewuski, a friend of the King who served as Poland's
envoy to St Petersburg. She belonged to the top Varsovian society and was
visited by representatives of the aristocracy as well as artists. The balls and parties
she threw were famous not only in the capital itself, but were also reported in
gazettes distributed out into the provinces, recounted in memoirs, and one
of her masquerades was even commemorated in verse.[17] Boruwłaski took part
in all of this, but did so as an underling of his benefactress rather than as an
independent figure, and so he writes little about it all. We know that he met the
newly-elected Polish King Stanisław Augustus and his brother Kazimierz. The
king was allegedly so enchanted with him that he wanted to take him under
his own protection, and Madame Geoffrin definitely wanted to take him away
to Paris,[18] but Boruwłaski does not mention these facts. In the later edition of
his memoirs he added that he had met the famous adventurer and swindler
Cagliostro at this time, and that is entirely possible – the latter was indeed in
Warsaw in 1780, enjoying vast but short-lived popularity among the highest
circles of Varsovian society. Certain doubts are only raised by his claim that
Cagliostro allegedly engaged himself in Joujou's romantic affairs at Countess
Humiecka's instigation.[19] Without any doubt, however, Boruwłaski did strike
up an acquaintance with Reichsgraf Stackelberg, the Russian ambassador to
Poland, who later even signed a subscription for his memoirs. We can surmise

---

[17]   J. Koblański, 'Oda na maski krakowskie w karnawał 1773 w bandzie J.W. Humieckiej,
Miecznikowej Koronnej', in *Wiersze Józefa Koblańskiego i Stanisława Szczęsnego Potockiego
zapomnianych poetów Oświecenia*, ed. E. Aleksandrowska, Wrocław, 1980, p. 70.

[18]   M.T. Geoffrin to Stanisław Augustus, 17 December 1770, in: *Correspondence inédité*,
p. 389.

[19]   J. Boruwlaski, *A Second Edition of the Memoirs of the Celebrated Dwarf, a Polish
Gentleman*, Birmingham, 1792 (cited hereinafter as *Memoirs* II), p. 69.

that in Countess Humiecka's salon he came into contact with all of Poland's elite society at that time, yet these events did not find any reflection in his memoirs.

That is not to say, however, that the passage of the memoirs dealing with the author's life in Warsaw is unexciting. On the contrary, it is extensive and considered the most interesting in the whole book. It undoubtedly represents the most personal fragment, and at the same time the best in terms of literary merit. It includes an account of Boruwłaski's early romance with a French starlet, which is interesting in and of itself, followed by the story of his love and marriage to Isalina Barboutan, presented in the form of love letters sent in both directions (although in reality there was perhaps love only in one direction, since the young lady's affections can be seriously doubted), originally written in French. Although the events presented in the memoirs really did take place, stirring up quite a sensation in Warsaw, his description of them is clearly written to comply with a certain literary concept, invoking the sentimental novel genre and portraying himself somewhat as the sentimental hero. He tells us of his emotional maturation, of his first 'worldly' love and painful disappointment, then of his profound and true affection for Isalina as the antithesis of his previous experience. Here we should note that Boruwłaski tried to follow the Enlightenment-age ideal of a relationship motivated by feelings rather than by propriety. It would be hard to imagine a marriage less conventional than his with Isalina, something he was well aware of. He begins the tale of his love by recounting his fears: 'It was not only the fear of becoming unacceptable to Isalina that dejected my mind. I apprehended that, should I succeed in winning her affection, could I engage her to lay aside prejudices, and be resolved concerning the union of her fate to mine, there would still remain many difficulties to overcome, either to gain her parents' consent, without which there was no hope left for me, or to obtain the sanction of my benefactress, who undoubtedly would think this marriage ridiculous, and by all means oppose it.' Then, like in a classical romance, comes a complication caused by the adversity of fate: in this case the resolute objection from Countess Humiecka, the benefactress of both, reluctant to accept the affections and especially the matrimonial plans of her little Joujou. The story thus proceeds through the forced separation of the lovers, a battle between despair and hope, a culminating moment when first Isalina and then Joujou are ousted from Humiecka's household, and finally the turning point: an intervention by Kazimierz Poniatowski, assistance from the king himself, and at long last a wedding in late 1779.

All of this is portrayed in Boruwłaski's letters to Isalina, which are of very fine literary merit. They represent the fragment of the memoirs that is most highly prized aesthetically for its beautiful form and distinct gracefulness, but at the same time it raises the most historical doubts. It has even been suggested that these letters were written *ex post facto* or that they might not have been written by Boruwłaski at all. It is hard to resolve this issue conclusively, especially since aside from one short and conventional letter to Charles James Fox we do not have any other text composed by Boruwłaski in French. However, there is one notable piece of circumstantial evidence indicating that the letters may indeed have been authentic: the fact that they do not portray the author of the memoirs in the best of light. Rather, they show that his affections were generally unrequited – Isalina clearly cannot imagine a marriage with him, writing back that she loves him as she would love a child but not as a man, and moreover it is evident that the marriage was forced upon her and she accepted it mainly because she had no other option. The attitude she signals in her letters almost clashes with the euphoria expressed by Boruwłaski after their union was cemented. If these letters had been artificially composed solely for the purposes of the book, surely they would have portrayed the author's situation more favourably? It seems that Boruwłaski even realised this himself, considering – a fact that has not yet been pointed out – that he cut this extensive correspondence out of the second edition of his memoirs, leaving just an assertion of their mutual affections and two letters which seem to confirm them. Following this line of reasoning, we may conclude that the letters are better written than the rest of the memoirs precisely because of their authenticity. In them the author does not attempt any stylistically elaborate constructions that fall somewhat flat, as he does elsewhere, but rather tries in simple fashion to voice his affections and the arguments in their defence. Another source of confirmation may be Boruwłaski's few preserved letters written in Polish, which are characterised by appalling spelling and unusual syntax but do have a certain charm attesting to their author's epistolary talents.

Although his own affections were undoubtedly authentic, we can nevertheless risk the assertion that not just Boruwłaski's description of his love, but even his entire attitude towards this period of his life constituted a kind of literary creation. In a certain sense, his love itself was more important to him than its object, whose resistance he was simply unwilling to recognise. Besides, later on, despite his praise of his wife's virtues, the memoirs do not tell us very much about her – mentions of her and their children mainly serve to underscore that despite his small stature, as the father of a family Boruwłaski was just as much a man as any other. Not much about her is known from other sources, either: her two preserved portraits, one by Frederic Anthony Lohrmann drawn up just after the wedding and the other an engraving by William Hincks published as the frontispiece of Boruwłaski's memoirs, portray her as a very pretty young woman, especially admired for her beautiful eyes. Born in 1762, she was 23 years younger than her husband, and her lively and cheerful disposition was stressed by Boruwłaski as well as outside observers. Catherine Hutton, who got to know her in England, wrote: 'She was of a middle size, very handsome and very lively; her dark eyes were particularly fine. She spoke English well and talked much and laughed and sang French songs,' going on to add: 'She was a woman whom any man might love, but certainly not a woman whom it was prudent for Boruwlaski to marry.'[20] Indeed, although every sentimental love-story should properly end at this point with a simple statement that the pair lived happily ever after, the Boruwłaskis' story in a certain sense was only now just beginning. In fact, they did not manage to stay together very long and their years together would not prove to be particularly happy.

---

[20]   C. Hutton, 'A Memoir of the Celebrated Dwarf Joseph Boruwlaski', *Bentley's Miscellany*, vol. 17, 1845, p. 247.

Chapter 2

An Involuntary Adventurer

Upon having left, or rather lost, his position serving Humiecka, Boruwłaski became an independent man for the first time in his life. But this was not a very autonomous sort of independence. His royal salary of 120 ducats proved to be insufficient for a married couple that had been accustomed to an affluent lifestyle, and especially so given their prospects for a rapidly growing family – their first child, a daughter, was born in January 1781. And so, following the persuasion of the King's brother, Boruwłaski decided to travel around the courts of Europe once again in order to entertain the world's great figures, this time on his own. In a certain sense he was choosing to take the path of the famous eighteenth-century adventurers. Just like them he became something of a citizen of the world, constantly changing location, possessing nothing and growing attached to nothing; just like them he tried to win the support of people from the highest strata, without actually himself fitting into the structure of eighteenth-century society. But the differences here are more distinct than the similarities. Such men as Casanova, Cagliostro, or their less well-known imitators consciously chose the fate of eternal wanderers, themselves remaining outside society; they concealed their true past and real origins; they avoided stabilisation, work, family. Boruwłaski's decisions, on the other hand, were made for him by nature and chance. He lived the life of an involuntary adventurer, one constantly trying to find a way out of the adventurer's lifestyle – and for a long time unsuccessfully so. His life for the next 25 years between 1780 and 1805 amounts to a ceaseless but futile attempt to find stabilisation, to find a place for himself in both the geographical and social senses. Such was the objective not only of his efforts to gain a stable income, but also of his stubbornly stressing that he was a Polish nobleman, the father of a family, in other words a man worthy of respect despite his oddity, one who deserved a certain place in society. Boruwłaski did not seek to blur his own past or origins; to the contrary for him they were an important element of his identity. Just how important is shown by the pride with which he stressed in his memoirs that the King of England had treated him not as 'an interesting curiosity' but as a Polish nobleman. Necessity had forced him to become perhaps not so much an adventurer as something along the lines of a peddler of his own body – although he never accepted that role and whenever he could he tried to liberate himself from it. This was not easy, because this role was something obvious to those around him, including his aristocratic 'benefactors.' They did not see anything wrong with the notion that a man whose sensitivity, intelligence, and high-society elegance they admired should put himself on display for money. They even considered it their duty to show him this as his rightful place, sometimes doing so quite brutally, like the French ambassador in Vienna, de Breteuil: 'you must needs give up pride, or choose misery; and if you do not intend to lead the most unhappy life; if you wish to enjoy, in future, a state of tranquillity, it is indispensable you should resolve to make exhibition of yourself.' Boruwłaski's account of the encounter continues: 'The next day the Prince de Kaunitz spoke to me in the same manner amidst a crowded levee.' He cites these comments in his memoirs without commentary, but from other of Boruwłaski's statements we can surmise that they must have come as substantial shocks to him. Especially since he probably was quietly hoping to find a permanent spot for himself in the household of some great lord or lady. For the first year of his travels he managed to avoid complying with that advice. As Kazimierz Poniatowski had anticipated, the German courts he visited still remembered his visit with Countess Humiecka, and his changed personal situation plus the romantic story of his love triggered considerable interest and a favourable reception. However, already then his predicament was quite strange – on the one hand he was received among the best society and monarchic courts, but on the other hand he lacked the money to meet his own basic needs. While still in Austria he tried to cope with this by giving numerous concerts. This, too, was essentially a form of exhibiting himself for money, but it was one he perceived as not as humiliating as what he would be forced to do later. In any event, he could believe, or at least tried to believe that the gathered audience was interested in his skill as a virtuoso – he did play both the guitar and violin quite well. Sometimes he was accompanied in these performances by professional musicians, like by the orchestra of the Count de Thüurheim or later in England by

Wilhelm Cramer, a member of the royal orchestra. Aside from that, these were events intended for a closed audience – mostly for high society, in view of both the price of the tickets (which in England was half a guinea, or more than the cost of supporting a modest family for a week) and the fact that most of them, sometimes all of them, were held among the circle of Boruwłaski's aristocratic protectors. He describes this custom in his memoirs, and in a surviving letter to Charles James Fox he persuades the prominent politician to buy tickets for his concert.[1] Such a performance still fit to some extent within the role he had been accustomed to, as a decoration and plaything of the salons. He would also exhibit himself together with his wife and sometimes children and relate his life story, but he was still doing so among the same type of people who had long been his audience – now they were just paying for it. Besides, they supported him financially in other ways as well. This portion of his memoirs is reminiscent of scrupulous accounting records, noting all the presents and gratification received from 'gracious benefactors': 30 ducats from the Countess Fekètè, a certain sum from the Elector of Bavaria, an ivory case from the Electress Dowager, a present of gold from the Prince de la Tour and Taxis, 40 luis-d'ors from the Margrave of Ansbach ... This list could be continued at length. Boruwłaski scrupulously tried to keep track of all his debts of gratitude – his memoirs were after all addressed to the givers of those presents, whom he did not want to and could not afford to slight by neglecting to mention them. On the other hand, this had an unfortunate impact on the concluding section of the memoirs' first edition, making it read somewhat like an accounting ledger. This was realised by the publisher of the second edition in 1792 who, despite the author's protests, removed most of these expressions of gratitude.[2]

The Boruwłaskis' voyage through Europe began in 1781 and took them first to Austria, then through Germany, where they visited several successive German princes, then through Strasbourg, Brussels, and Ostend, and then onward to England, where they arrived in March 1782. It is worth pointing out immediately that in the fourth and final edition of his memoirs, dating from 1820, Boruwłaski paints a completely different picture of his voyage ('his' because he no longer

---

[1]   J. Boruwłaski to Charles James Fox, 9 June 1783 (British Library, MS Add. 47563, p. 151).

[2]   *Memoirs* II, introduction, p. xxix.

mentions his wife and children), embellishing this particular period of his life to an astonishing degree. He claims to have been not just in Austria and Germany, but also to have allegedly travelled through Hungary, Turkey, Russia, all the way up to Finland and Lapland, across all of Siberia to the Arctic Ocean and the Bering Strait, then making a return journey through Bukhara, Croatia, and Dalmatia, not to mention an excursion to the Mediterranean Sea, visiting Tunisia, and going looking for the philosopher's stone there together with the Hungarian explorer and adventurer Maurice Benyowsky. Setting aside for the time being the issue of why these voyages suddenly appeared in the memoirs and what function the tales served, we need to categorically assert that none of them actually took place and of all the locations mentioned Boruwłaski in fact visited only Hungary at the invitation of the Countess Fekètè. In the final edition of his memoirs, the author cautiously avoids giving any dates – and rightfully so, because all this alleged travelling is said to have lasted more than three years, and under no circumstances could it have fit between February 1781 and March 1782. These are the known dates of his departure from Poland and his arrival to England, which were stated down to the day in the first edition of the memoirs and confirmed by outside sources, chiefly the press.[3]

The account of the trip from Poland to England also raises another mysterious issue, one that is not as easy to settle so categorically. Although in his memoirs Boruwłaski tries to give the impression that they travelled alone and that as head of the family he bore sole responsibility for the comfort and safety of his wife and child, in reality the Boruwłaskis did have a fellow traveller who took care of the whole family. This is quite a shadowy figure, mentioned in the memoirs essentially only once at the very end, where the author regrets that he will probably lose the 'friendship and counsels of a generous man, who, through regard for distinguished persons my protectors in Poland, has been so kind as to accompany me in my travels.' This generous man was a certain de Trouville, about whom we unfortunately know very little. In Catherine Hutton's memoirs he appears as an uncle of Isalina (perhaps we should more safely write

---

[3]   This was pointed out by H.R. Heatley, the English publisher of the supplemented memoirs in 1902, noting that 'it is impossible to insert these years between February 11, 1781 and March 20, 1782' – suggesting that these descriptions resulted from poor memory and problems in communicating with the translator. *The Life and Love Letters...*, p. 95, publisher's note.

'uncle' in quotation marks here, although Hutton herself does not question the relation outright). It seems that he accompanied the Boruwłaskis in their travels all the way until 1787. A letter written by Joseph in Dublin to Polish minister in London Franciszek Bukaty indicates that his duties included that of an impresario, handling negotiations on the organisation of concerts.[4] It is not clear precisely when their parting of ways, which the author of the memoirs later expresses such regret about, actually occurred or what may have triggered it. His writings indicate that it was prompted by the intervention of third parties, who deemed de Trouville's company to be harmful to Boruwłaski.

The Boruwłaskis' journey through Germany, which lasted more than a year, was not extraordinarily eventful. Successive rulers of the German statelets sent them onward to their crowned cousins and relatives, together with letters of recommendation that ensured them a warm reception. The visits played out in similar fashion: a first audience at the court that enraptured all those assembled, invitations for another visit or several visits, often a concert for the local aristocracy, receiving a present from the prince, and ... a voyage onward. Boruwłaski did not manage to acquire what he was presumably most anxiously seeking – a stable position at one of the courts. He only managed to secure a future for his first daughter – Ansbach's ruling couple took the infant under their care, promising to look after her welfare. An apostrophe addressed to this abandoned daughter which he includes in his memoirs seems to serve as a kind of public reminder to them of their promises.

It was already in Vienna, under the influence of the representative of Great Britain to Austria, Sir Robert Keith, that the Boruwłaskis decided that England would be the ultimate destination of their journey. The ambassador not only praised the wealth and kindness of his country's inhabitants, but also outfitted Boruwłaski with letters of recommendation to the highest-ranking aristocrats in the land, to which were added letters from Chancellor Kaunitz

---

4   'J.W. Mci Pana Ruspiniego, zaś w loży gdy była rozmowa Pana Ruspiniego z panem detruvillem zglendem grania na gitarze, rozumiem aby do niego napisał, ponieważ z nim o wszystkim traktował' ['As for Mr Ruspini, as there was a conversation in the theatre-box between Mr Ruspini and Mr Detruville concerning guitar-playing, I believe he should write to him because he had negotiated everything with him']. J. Boruwłaski to F. Bukaty, Dublin, 29 Oct. 1784, Archiwum Główne Akt Dawnych [Polish Central Archives of Historical Records] (cited hereinafter as AGAD), Zbiory Muzeum Naodowego [National Museum Collection], 79).

and later the Margrave Ansbach, among others. Indeed, the addressees of those recommendations were individuals who could ensure Boruwłaski access to the very highest society, and more importantly actually did so. Without a doubt the most valuable acquaintance proved to be Georgiana, Duchess of Devonshire; he had probably received suggestions of this in advance since she was the first member of high society which he approached arriving in London. The 25-year-old Georgiana Devonshire herself came from the prominent Spencer family, and in 1774 she had married the best match in the kingdom, William Cavendish, Duke of Devonshire. She quickly became the unparalleled queen of London high society. Although her extravagance, affectation, and political involvement were ridiculed, at the same time she was a target of much admiration and interest. Her salon near Piccadilly was frequented by politicians, scholars, and writers.[5] Boruwłaski's memoirs are far from unique in describing her as a good-natured, kind woman eager to help those in need. Her kindness was quite simply invaluable to Boruwłaski in the initial stage of his sojourn in the British Isles, since apart from her generous financial support the Duchess recommended him to practically 'everyone who was anyone' in London. Suffice it to mention that her acquaintances included the Prince of Wales and that her mother was Georgiana Spencer, a lady nearly just as influential and at the same time famous for her generosity (a trait important to Boruwłaski). It is not surprising that the first concert Boruwłaski gave at Carlisle House in Soho on 31 May 1782 proved to be a great success. We can surmise this was partly due to his visit with King George III, which had been reported in the newspapers. And so Boruwłaski had become fashionable yet again, only this time in England. He was once again invited to the most exclusive salons and entertained elegant society. While it is true that baroque notions akin to serving him to table in an urn were no longer acted out (besides, he was now too large for such shenanigans, having grown to his 'full' 99 centimetres), his role had still essentially not changed very much. This is evidenced by the meeting arranged by his aristocratic friends between him and Charles Byrne, the young 'Irish Giant' who was nearly two

---

[5]   A thorough biography of the Duchess was published by Amanda Foreman: *Georgiana, Duchess of Devonshire*, 1st edn, HarperCollins, 1998.

and a half metres tall. This meeting between two opposite freaks of nature was even reported in the press.[6]

This was therefore to a certain extent a repeat of Boruwłaski's success from the years of his youth. However, his situation was different than it had been, and England under George III was certainly not the same as France under Louis XV. Aside from that, the rapture of the world at large was something very ephemeral, the fashion for the little Pole did not last much longer than a year in London, and Boruwłaski needed a stable income to support the costs of his family rather than just occasional (albeit initially quite sizeable) assistance from the aristocracy. Especially since those costs were not small, estimated by the author at 400–500 pounds a year. That is a sizeable sum, if one considers that the Polish poet and traveller Julian Ursyn Niemcewicz living in London at the same period paid a guinea and a half per week (which comes to around 82 pounds per year) for a fully serviced apartment in a good location.[7] Boruwłaski quite convincingly explained the reason for his relatively high expenses – he essentially did not have any stable place of residence, which given his unfamiliarity with English realities surely increased his costs considerably, as did his frequent trips, the organisation of concerts (renting out venues, paying accompanying musicians, advertising, and so on), and also his family was again growing larger – a second daughter, Georgiana Fanny (known in Polish as 'Franusia') was born in May 1783, and a third was probably born at the end of 1784 during his stay in Ireland.[8]

Boruwłaski dreamed of obtaining a single larger sum of money that would enable him to lead an independent life, but attempts made by his protectors

---

[6]   *Morning Post*, 30 May 1782.

[7]   J.U. Niemcewicz, *Pamiętniki czasów moich*, ed. J. Dihm, Warszawa 1957, p. 229

[8]   While the birth of the second daughter was announced in the *Morning Herald* on 6 May 1783 ('Yesterday morning was delivered of a girl, the Lady of Comte Boruwlaski, the wonderful dwarf of Polish Russia'), the third's arrival, as suggested in the memoirs, is confirmed by Catherine Hutton's account that in December 1785 the Boruwłaskis had two children: a somewhat elder girl and a breastfeeding infant (C. Hutton, op. cit., p. 47). Boruwłaski mentions the Polish name of his second daughter in a letter to Franciszek Bukaty from Dublin, 29 Oct. 1784 (AGAD, Zbiory Muzeum Narodowego, 79), whereas her full names are listed on the tombstone at Montmartre cemetery in Paris: 'Georgiana Fanny Boruwlaska, veuve Kean, née à Londres le 6 mai 1783 décédée à Paris le 29 décembre 1856' – recorded by Maurice Devos.

several times to take up a collection all failed and he was left with no option but to earn money by making a spectacle of himself before an audience that was gradually growing less and less refined. He sensed this as something humiliating, as is confirmed by the way he mentions it in the first edition of his memoirs, and demonstrated even more prominently by the fact that he omitted all reference to this aspect of his life in the subsequent edition. In a certain sense he thus fit into the whole, highly diverse group of people entertaining various spheres of English society in those days. The demand for such entertainment was great, but this was generally a very short-lived kind of celebrity, necessitating constant changing of location. The general competition in the field was also considerable, and even in terms of individuals his own size Boruwłaski faced a number of rivals advertised in the press: a Peter Bono (3 feet and several inches) was selling a small portrait of himself for half a pence, bearing a short dedication for the nobility and gentry, a Miss Morgan and Mr Allen regularly drew public attention in 1781–1791, a miniature Miss Purte advertised herself in 1787, followed by Joseph Cordero several years later. And apart from them there were of course many others: giants, bearded women, wild-men – such as Indian 'warriors' or the African lion-tamer Macomo – plus a whole slew of charlatans exhibiting miraculous inventions, and many, many other performers ranging all the way to tightrope-walkers and clowns (such as the famous Grimaldi), not mention even tamed wild animals. Boruwłaski was fully aware of his predicament. Years later, when he was able to approach this with a sense of distance, he wrote with bitter irony about his first stay in Bath in the winter of 1782/1783: 'I had not been long there, before the arrival of the learned pig was announced in that city. The proprietor of that wonderful animal, bringing with him from London strong recommendations of its abilities, attracted crowded audiences of all the gentry; so that I thought it most prudent to return to London.'[9]

Contrary to the suggestions of certain authors, to the best of our knowledge Boruwłaski never had to exhibit himself to the masses at public market squares. He offered, so to speak, more elegant forms of entertainment, intended for a somewhat more affluent audience. We have already mentioned his concerts, which were profitable ventures insofar as an audience turned out in good numbers, but they also required considerable outlays – the amount of 80

---

[9]   *Memoirs* IV, p. 188.

guineas mentioned in the memoirs for organising a concert in London was a vast sum, hence such concerts took place relatively rarely, at most once in a given town or city. An equally serious type of venture involved balls thrown by Boruwłaski – in his memoirs he describes one such ball given in Dublin. Not all of them enjoyed the kind of illustrious patronage as the one in Dublin (from the Lord Lieutenant of Ireland), not all of them were opened by a duke and duchess, but they all followed a similar scheme. A surviving advertisement describes all the attractions that awaited anyone prepared to pay the 5 shilling entrance fee for an event organised by Boruwłaski on 30 May 1788 at the 'Crown and Anchor' inn on the Strand in London. The ball lasted from 8.00 p.m. until 1.00 a.m. Boruwłaski entertained his guests with conversation and above all with performances. He played the guitar as usual, but it seems he sparked greater interest with the Cossack dance he performed together with his wife – a performance the *Morning Herald* charmingly reported that Vestris, the most famous dancer of the time, would not have been ashamed of. After his encores, the ball proper would begin and the host would dance with the ladies present.[10] From Boruwłaski's perspective there was nothing insulting in this, he was simply the thrower of a party, a 'host' graciously entertaining his guests. The public breakfasts he often gave were of a somewhat similar character. In his memoirs he writes about one such event in Bath, a highly successful one judging by the number of tickets sold. Like in the case of the paid-attendance balls, Boruwłaski did not treat this as his making a humiliating spectacle of his small size. As one witness of his stay in Scotland commented: 'The Count did not, at least in Edinburgh, exhibit himself as a dwarf – indeed his feelings would not have allowed of such a thing – he merely "received company." He gave a public breakfast, to participate at which the small charge of 3s. 6d. was demanded.'[11] As in other cases, here the host entertained his guests with his guitar and above all his scintillating conversation. He must have been a charming speaker indeed, because the English accounts of Boruwłaski, like the surviving commentaries from the years of his youth, are full of rapture at his intellect and refinement: the same Scottish writer summed him up as 'a person of cultivated mind and

---

[10]   *Morning Herald*, 29 May 1788, ball announcement; *Morning Herald*, 2 June 1788, follow-up report on the ball.

[11]   *A Series of Original Portraits and Caricature Etchings, by late John Kay [...] with Biographical Sketches and Illustrative Anecdotes*, vol.1, Edinburgh, 1837, p. 329.

possessed of high conversational powers.'[12] But note that at least through the first few years in Britain the virtues of his conversation could only have been appreciated by highly educated audiences, since he must have been speaking French. When landing in the British Isles Boruwłaski did not know English at all and found it difficult to learn, unlike his wife, who quickly began to speak the language with ease. In fact he would never learn the language entirely well – to the constant amusement of the English, whose recollections of him recount with relish how he distorted English grammar or especially pronunciation. With time, this would become something of an advantage for him. As his friend Charles Mathews wrote, these humorous linguistic mistakes, in conjunction with his bright intellect and wit, gave his speeches a special charm and allure.[13] Initially, however, this shortcoming must have posed quite an obstacle for a man whose main talent was witty conversation.

While such paid-entrance concerts, balls, and even breakfasts enabled him to preserve at least outward appearances that the 'guests' were motivated by a desire for entertainment, rather than just ordinary curiosity, the paid visits that were offered to Boruwłaski's apartment left no doubt that the drawing point was simply his unusual physique. Despite his reluctance to resort to taking such visits, he was ultimately forced to do so relatively quickly. From at least the winter of 1783, he exhibited himself at his apartment at 29 St James Street for 5 shillings, every day from noon to 3.00 p.m. and from 6.00 to 9.00 p.m. A 'special' visit to someone else's home could also be arranged at a higher price – half a guinea for each guest involved. Boruwłaski was quite soon forced to lower these prices to one shilling per normal visit to his home and half a crown (2.5 shillings) per special visit; the latter price would remain in place almost until the end of his 'career.'[14] In every location where he stayed he placed announcements in the press and sometimes also printed pamphlets, presumably to be pasted on walls and also tossed onto the doorsteps of homes, announcing that the given town

---

[12]   Ibidem, p. 330.

[13]   *Memoirs of Charles Mathews Comedian*, by Ann Mathews, London, 1839, vol. 3, p. 218.

[14]   At the very end its price rose to 2 shillings, probably in connection with a general inflation of prices, but also because Boruwłaski was exhibiting himself in London after a 15-year interval and was probably hoping for a resurgence of interest. Cf. *Morning Herald*, 24 Jan. 1805.

was being visited by the famous dwarf from Polish Russia who was inviting the public to come and see 'the most astonishing curiosity sportive nature ever held out to admiration of mankind' – as one poster from Bristol lauded him.[15] From the advertising standpoint, it was most effective when such an announcement preceded a concert or ball – at such times interest in Boruwłaski surged and those who could not afford to attend the expensive event itself could satisfy their curiosity by visiting him at his home. We do not know much about these visits. The author himself generally avoids describing them; the last edition of the memoirs makes more frequent reference to them but there he usually tries to give the impression that these were normal social calls. He is said to have told his friends years later that he merely extended his hospitality to guests who came to his home, and it was their business if they gave his butler a shilling to let them in: 'I receive de visets and peopul give my valet shilling for open the door' – Catherine Hutton reports him as saying, trying to give her readers an impression of the way he spoke English.[16] During these visits he did indeed try to recreate the aura of the elegant banter of the salons, something that was appreciated by at least some of those visiting him; he later struck up lasting acquaintances with many of them and was invited to their homes not as a freak-show, but as a charming guest – or as one of his hosts described it: 'he always proved if not a great addition [to the assembled company] then at least a pleasing one.'[17] However, we can surmise that quite often he was exposed to treatment that bruised his ego, or even affronted his sense of dignity. Catherine Hutton, who as a small girl got to know him while visiting his home in Birmingham, recalled him as a sad and taciturn man – the latter attribute presumably due to his still poor English.[18] However, we should point out that Boruwłaski's sense of humour was an important part of his character and moreover we should not forget about his years of attendance at the world's top salons, where conversation was always based upon a light exchange of opinions and compliments, but also the ability to

---

[15]   Leaflet dated 25 Aug. 1783, in D. Lyson, *Lyson's colletanea, or a collection of advertisement and paragraphs from the newspapers relating to various subjects, vol. 1: Public exhibitions and places of amusement.*

[16]   C. Hutton, op. cit., p. 48.

[17]   *A Series of Original Portraits*, p. 330.

[18]   This meeting occurred in December 1785, and the Boruwłaskis were later guests in the home of Catherine's father, where they spent Christmas. C. Hutton, op. cit., p. 247.

make witty retorts. These character traits presumably earned him popularity and sympathy, and also enabled him to cope with various types of tactless boors. The remarks he had to suffer from such people were not always related to his size. In his memoirs he recalls a discussion with a certain overweight lady who, having found out that he was a Catholic, voiced her doubt about whether he would make it into heaven. Boruwłaski responded by citing the biblical reference to the narrow gate of heaven, then glanced at her girth and added that he thought he himself stood a much better chance of squeezing through such an entranceway.[19] We can surmise that most of the guests were nevertheless not interested in Boruwłaski's personality but in his odd physique, and some people were quite simply brutal in how they vented their curiosity. One interesting event was described in the *Morning Herald* in March 1786: a certain young man attended a visit to Boruwłaski's apartment in the Strand and soon after arriving began to inquire, with ridicule and mockery, about Boruwłaski's wife who happened to be absent and about his children, generally suggesting doubts that the host could actually have a normal family. Eventually he even called into question his capabilities as a man. Boruwłaski initially tried to deal with the situation elegantly, asking this nuisance about his own marriage and asking him to refer to his host's capabilities in this regard with the same respect as to his own. Finally, irritated at the guest's continued mockery and openly expressed doubt at whether Isalina could possibly be content with him, Boruwłaski turned to the guest to make the following proposal: 'whatever either I or my wife might say on this subject, would not remove your doubts. I know but one method of giving you complete satisfaction; you say you are married; your wife is, doubtless handsome.' The guest assented, and Boruwłaski continued: 'Why, then, if you will permit me to pass the night with her, I will engage, that tomorrow morning, she will be perfectly mistress of the point in dispute, and be fully enabled to answer all questions.' It is no surprise that upon hearing this, the boor simply walked out.[20] This account is especially valuable in that it was not penned years after the fact by Boruwłaski in his memoirs, but shortly after the incident itself, most likely by someone highly amused at the scene he had witnessed.

---

[19]　*Memoirs* IV, p. 197.
[20]　*Morning Herald*, 11 Mar. 1786.

'Most likely' because most of the press reports about Boruwłaski were in fact published for advertising purposes, written at the behest of and probably paid for by Boruwłaski himself. From the very beginning of his stay in England, presumably at the advice and with the assistance of either one of his English protectors or de Trouville, he availed himself widely of the advertising possibilities offered by the British press, which was then much more modern than the continental press. Aside from the above-mentioned announcements inviting guests to his concerts, balls, breakfasts, and home visits, the press carried follow-up summaries of those events and sometimes also quite sizeable articles about Boruwłaski and his life story – such as a whole-column article in the *Gazetteer* in 1786, quoting fragments Count de Tressan's report on him further supplemented to cover the interim years of Boruwłaski's life.[21] Similarly, when his memoirs were being prepared for print subscription, teaser advertisements first appeared in many newspapers, followed by announcements of the book's publication, and afterwards certain dailies even carried reviews or large summaries.[22] The fact that Boruwłaski appreciated the importance of advertising is shown by the gratefulness he expresses in the 1820 edition of the memoirs to a certain Mr Walker, who had helped him in Newcastle in 1801 by having several thousand concert posters printed at his own cost, and also by paying for newspaper advertisements, which was not something cheap.[23]

Just by following the surviving mentions of Boruwłaski in the press, one can very nearly trace out on the map the route of his travels through Great Britain – which all in all lasted 20 years. Not quite a year after arriving in the country, he had already left London in the winter of 1782/1783 for a short trip to follow his aristocratic audience to Bath. He undertook a larger journey to Ireland in early August 1783 (not in April as he writes in his memoirs), along the way exhibiting himself in Bristol (a preserved announcement of this is dated 25 August) and in Chester. In Ireland, where he also took his wife and child, he spent more than two years and his third daughter was born. In December 1785 he was once again in England, although it was not until March 1786 that he returned to London, where he settled for more than two years. In his memoirs, or at least in their first

---

[21] *Gazetteer*, 19 Oct. 1786.

[22] *Morning Herald*, 29 May 1788, a review encouraging purchase; *Bath Chronicle*, 7 Aug. 1788, an extensive summary.

[23] *Memoirs* IV, p. 350.

edition, he limits himself exclusively to mentioning the kind reception he was given in all the places he visited by people among the highest social circles, most often the aristocracy. But he does not mention the hardships of day-to-day life, the inconveniences of travel, all the uncomfortable trains, greedy innkeepers, or inclement weather he must have had to endure (only once does he vent his bitterness at a dishonest servant and his resulting feeling of powerlessness). Presumably he thought that such things would be of little interest to his refined readers. Certain mentions of this sort, although also brief and generally written in a jocular tone, appear only in the last edition of the memoirs. But to fully realise the difficulties Boruwłaski had to face, one has to recall that he had spent his whole early life under the care of the Countess Humiecka, essentially without any contact with any of the nuisances of daily life. Hence his complete lack of experience, which at least initially made him easy prey for various swindlers and con-artists. He described one of them, an alleged 'Marquis de Montpellier,' in his memoirs but this was not his only encounter of the sort. He more frequently encountered petty swindlers operating on a smaller scale than this 'marquis,' but all in all they were probably even more of a nuisance to him – all the dishonest innkeepers and greedy entrepreneurs. He summed this up nicely in his memoirs, when describing how one such gentleman had organised a concert for him: this man was so good at arithmetic, especially at division, that in the final tally he received the money from the event, whereas Boruwłaski received figures on a paper.[24] It seems that for the first few years after leaving Poland Boruwłaski was protected from such contacts to a significant degree by de Trouville, but after the latter's departure around 1788, Boruwłaski was already left solely to his own devices.

We can conjecture that after their return from Ireland the Boruwłaskis were tired of travelling; in any case they did make an attempt at staying in the capital for good. But their situation was not easy, aristocratic society already seems to have grown a bit weary of Joseph, audience turnout at his concerts and balls was not the best, and even worse, for some time now his stipend from Polish King Stanisław Augustus had ceased to arrive. In 1788 he still made an attempt, via Tadeusz Bukaty the cousin and deputy of Franciszek Polish chargé d'affaires, to

---

[24]   Ibidem, p. 218.

seek its reinstatement, but generally to no avail.[25] Boruwłaski ended up in debt, facing the prospect of serious trouble or even imprisonment, and was rescued by the Princess Lubomirska, who then happened to be in London.

It was at this time that the idea of publishing his memoirs arose. The book was meant to stoke up interest in Boruwłaski, to remind powerful protectors of his existence, and subscriptions to the memoirs would also give the author a financial boost. Initially he intended to dedicate them to King Stanisław Augustus,[26] but given the king's objection he decided upon a dedication to his current protectress, the Duchess of Devonshire. The memoirs appeared in 1788 in a bilingual version, in French and English, so as to make them accessible to the broadest possible audience. Their publication can be considered a success – more than 400 individuals were on the subscription list, including all of Boruwłaski's aristocratic acquaintances from both London and Dublin, even the English heir to the throne and the royal family. That success is confirmed by the republication of the memoirs just four years later, sparking no less interest, as is shown by the equally long (albeit less aristocratic) list of individuals eager to buy them. Aside from the volumes meant for subscribers, Boruwłaski also offered the book for sale to visitors who came to see his home, as noted in his press advertisements. The memoirs were soon translated into German as well. In all, the book undoubtedly sustained his fame and even made him into a certain point of reference. An announcement in the Berlin press in 1799, describing the chance to witness the tiny Nanette Stockbrin, compared her height and virtues to those of Boruwłaski.[27]

The profits from the memoirs were not sufficient to cover Boruwłaski's expenses for very long, hence the need arose for a new voyage, which he embarked

---

[25]   T. Bukaty to the Department of Foreign Interests of the Permanent Council, London, 27 May 1788 (AGAD, Archiwum Królestwa Polskiego [Archives of the Kingdom of Poland], 82, sheet 280). This letter reports that Boruwłaski had not been receiving his royal stipend for several years.

[26]   The announcement of the subscription in the *Morning Post* states that the memoirs would be dedicated to the King of Poland. Stanisław Augustus sharply protested: 'W. Pan napisz, żeby on temu Boruwłaskiemu powiedział ode mnie, żeby on mi tego swego życia nie dedykował.' ['Write to Bukaty to tell that Boruwłaski from me that he should not dedicate that life of his to me.'] Stanisław Augustus to Pius Kiciński, 24 Feb. 1787 (Czartoryski Library, manuscript 924, sheet 389).

[27]   E.J. Wood, op. cit., London 1868, p. 395.

upon in 1788. This time it led northward, first to Cambridge, Norwich, and Bury St Edmunds, then on to Scotland, which Boruwłaski reached in early August of that year, as is shown by an announcement from Edinburgh about a breakfast he held. His reception in Scotland must have been very favourable, judging by the recollections left behind by Edinburgh residents and by mentions in Boruwłaski's own memoirs. Already in the 1792 edition, his stay in Scotland is depicted concisely but very warmly. Boruwłaski's subsequent visits to the country seem to have been similarly successful; we know that he was there again in 1802, appearing in public but also being received quite warmly by high society – he was the guest of General John Dickinson and his son, Captain Archibald.[28] It is not surprising that years later, to some extent provoked by Samuel Johnson's critical evaluation of the Scots, Boruwłaski undertook to defend them in his memoirs, admiring not only their courtesy but also their thriftiness and high intellectual level, not to mention the charm and beauty of Scottish women.[29]

Such remarks lead us to pose the broader question of what kind of circles Boruwłaski actually moved in. If we are to believe the first and second editions of his memoirs, he fraternised exclusively with the aristocratic elite. This picture is perhaps not false, but definitely one-sided. In his first years on the British Isles, Boruwłaski certainly did enjoy great popularity among the highest circles of English society. That is confirmed by the subscription list for the first edition of the memoirs, which does not lack nearly any British surname that carried any weight at the time, mostly those of noble blood but also those of significant politicians including Charles James Fox and the Lord Thomas Townshend. As in the years of his youth, Boruwłaski entertained such refined society with his personality and conversation. He presumably felt good in this role, which he had played for many years and always strove to perform as best he could. Indeed, he considered it his duty. As he writes following his audience with the British royal family: 'having used all my efforts to please them, I enjoyed the satisfaction of seeing that, in some respect, I had not failed in my aim.' His aristocratic protectors passed him off to one another as a pleasant form of short-lived entertainment. Letters of recommendation led him along his trips,

---

[28]   *The Memoirs of Susan Sibbald (1783–1812)*, ed. by her great-grandson Francis Paget Hett, London, 1926, p. 145.

[29]   *Memoirs* IV, p. 213–216.

assuring him a good reception not just in London but also throughout England, Ireland, and Scotland. However, despite what the memoirs seem to indicate, even during the period of the greatest interest in Boruwłaski, his contacts with the aristocracy were more episodic than stable and as interest waned over time they become increasingly rare. But at the same time we also know that he made a great many acquaintances, sometimes lasting and sometimes fleeting, among circles far removed from the aristocracy. However, no trace of them can be found in the first edition of the memoirs. It is telling to compare two descriptions of the Boruwłaski family's arrival to London in 1781. The account in the earlier memoirs begins straight away with a visit to the Duchess of Devonshire, in a way that suggests Boruwłaski headed in her direction immediately after reaching the capital city. The memoirs published years later, however, indicate that this was not the case, that he and his family initially stayed with and were warmly received by a certain Mr MacMahon, to whom he had been recommended by another Irishman met back in Brussels, a Mr Mills. This was not the only belated debt of gratitude the author repaid years after the fact – many previously omitted names resurface in the last edition of the memoirs. Some of his acquaintances are also known to us from third-party accounts. In the initial years of his stay in England, Boruwłaski maintained quite close contacts with the Poles there: aside from his 'benefactors' he mentions in the memoirs, Michał Kazimierz Ogiński and Izabela Lubomirska, and apart from individuals met by chance, like the writer Julian Ursyn Niemcewicz or the poet and traveller Kajetan Węgierski, whom he encountered in Ireland, he was above all on friendly terms with the brothers Franciszek and Tadeusz Bukaty, Polish diplomatic representatives in London, who repeatedly assisted him with various problems. But be that as it may, his main circle of acquaintances was decidedly English. This was a very broad circle, as Boruwłaski's way of life forced him to maintain contacts with a great many people from highly varied domains. It was customary that during his stay in a given town, after presenting himself to the public, he would spend the evenings with a family that wished to host him. This was how the family of Catherine Hutton, who wrote recollections of him years later, got to know him more closely. He undoubtedly had a gift of easily making acquaintances, skill at adapting to nearly every company. This flexibility of Boruwłaski is all the more surprising in that essentially until the age of 40 he had moved exclusively among the elite world of salons, without having practically any contact with other circles of society. And yet during his trip around Great Britain he proved just as capable of having a pleasant chat with the Prince of Wales as with a chance table-mate at a roadside inn, he felt just as at home in the salons of the Duke of Marlborough as in a military garrison off somewhere in provincial Ireland. He was – as he writes about himself, and as is confirmed by numerous witnesses – an open, amiable, and cheerful man, which undoubtedly helped him forge new acquaintances and friendships. He was also a refined and experienced man, this presumably underlying his numerous acquaintances among people in the free professions (lawyers, doctors) and also among merchants, clergymen, and military officers. The artist John Key immortalised in an engraving a walk Boruwłaski once took with one such acquaintance, the lawyer Neil Fergusson, along the streets of Edinburgh. Many of those acquaintances appear in the last edition of the memoirs, including such well-known figures as the prominent scientist Thomas Hope, a professor of chemistry and medicine at Edinburgh University; the inventor Matthew Boulton; General George Nuget, the commander of the English troops in Northern Ireland; and Reynold Gideon Bouyer, the archdeacon of Northumberland. However, a vast majority of their names were never recorded for history. These were frequently fleeting acquaintances, but sometimes turned into lasting affections. Boruwłaski enjoyed such affection from the five Metcalfe sisters: Sophia, Emma, Margaret, and two others known to us only by their initials ('J.' and 'L.'). We do not know precisely what kind of circles they moved in, but they were undoubtedly from a very wealthy and respected family – perhaps related to Thomas Metcalfe, director of the British East India Company, although this is nothing more than conjecture. This acquaintance, forged already in 1783, lasted until the end of the ladies' lives. Boruwłaski visited them at their rural estate in Bury St Edmunds, and then in London as late as the 1820s. Indeed, although their friendship brought him quite tangible benefits, it does seem that he especially appreciated the personal kindness they showed him, above all the fact that they treated him like a normal person. His heart was probably particularly won over by the fact that when his aristocratic benefactors were persuading him to abandon his scruples about putting himself on public display, the Metcalfe sisters found the idea revolting and scandalous[30] – and this was more than just empty talk on their part, as we will soon see.

One more professional group is worth pointing out, whose representatives Boruwłaski would maintain especially long-lasting bonds of friendship with: actors. During his lifelong journeying, Joseph met most of the outstanding actors of his epoch. While he did not manage to persuade the famous Mrs Siddons to grace his concert with her presence, the just as famous Wright and Monro did attend his appearances in Newcastle.[31] It is not clear when he got to know the brother of Mrs Siddons, Stephen Kemble, a Shakespearean actor somewhat less well known than his sister, but we do know that they became close friends. Finally, during his wanderings he got to know Charles Mathews the elder, one of the best known comic actors of the day, who not only shared a lifelong friendship with Boruwłaski (to the end of Mathews' life – Boruwłaski outlived most of his acquaintances) but also wrote one of the most extensive recollections of Joseph. In all his closer relations with actors were presumably facilitated by an affinity of roles, since after all both they and he put themselves on show to the public for money, and so once Boruwłaski's actor acquaintances grew accustomed to his oddity he became for them something of a professional colleague rather than a freak or wonder.

Essentially it is not clear whether the Boruwłaskis went to Scotland as a whole family, or whether Joseph went on his own. It seems likely that Isalina stayed behind in London, perhaps expecting another child. The introduction to the 1792 edition of the memoirs speaks of four Boruwłaski children (including the 11-year-old daughter who had remained in Ansbach). In fact, this is the last information that appears about the current state of his family. The 1792 edition does still mention his wife and children, although much less often and more concisely than in the first edition. And Isalina disappears almost completely from the last edition of 1820. We do not learn anything about her beyond the abbreviated story of Joujou's love for her, essential for motivating subsequent events, and he does not speak of his family at all. Insofar as he mentioned his wife at all after 1792, Boruwłaski tried to suggest that he was a widower.[32]

---

[30] Ibidem, p. 190.

[31] Ibidem, p. 349.

[32] Such information from 1802 was found by Tom Heron, op. cit., p. 17; a report of his wife's death was also provided in *Biographia Curiosa or Memoirs of Remarkable Characters of*

Judging by the commentaries he made the few times he did mention her, he did not remember her fondly. An epitaph-in-verse he once recited during his audience with George IV, when asked about the fate of his wife, is indicative: '*Ci git ma femme. Ah! qu'elle est bien,/Pour son repos, et pour le mien.*' (Here lieth my wife. How good that be/for the peaceful rest of her – and me).[33] In fact, this quipping couplet was highly appreciated by the king, unable to bear his own wife, Caroline of Brunswick, with whom he had been separated for years yet was unable to secure parliamentary consent to divorce her. But Boruwłaski was not in fact a widower. His marriage had most probably fallen apart, though it is not clear under what circumstances the couple had actually fallen out. Catherine Hutton writes that when she met him again in 1792, Joseph was already alone.[34] It seems that we should trace the break-up to the trip to Ireland in 1792.

But before that, Boruwłaski had made one more voyage in 1790. This has been mistakenly identified by some authors as a trip to Poland,[35] but in fact it was to France, along the way calling at Bath and Bristol again. This was a very unsuccessful trip. Not only was his health giving him trouble, and not only did he fall prey to a con-man who stole his money, but Boruwłaski reached the country in the spring of 1790 and Paris itself in June, thus arriving in the very middle of revolution. It is ironic that it was precisely on 19 June 1790, almost at the very moment of his arrival to Paris, that the National Constituent Assembly announced the abolition of the nobility. And so, the very stratum of society whose curiosity ensured Boruwłaski a way to make a living officially ceased to exist. It was not yet eradicated physically, as this would not start to actually happen to representatives of the nobility until some two years later, but its concerns and passions were definitely different than in years gone by. Although the names of Boruwłaski's old acquaintances do appear in the memoirs – the Marquis d'Amazaga, the Duchess of Orleans – but the interest he sparked was

---

the *Reign of George the Third*, collected by George Smeeton and others, London 1822, p. 79 – which was published during Boruwłaski's lifetime.

[33]   *Memoirs of Charles Mathews*, p. 220.

[34]   C. Hutton, op. cit., p. 247 ff.

[35]   *The New Wonderful Museum*, ed. William Granger, London, 1804, p. 1076; Henry Wilson, *Wonderful Characters*, vol. 3, London, 1822, p. 389; Edward J. Wood, op. cit., p. 342. All these authors give the date of the trip at 1792 rather than 1790, but they do not note the earlier trip at all, which gives rise to the suspicion that a double mistake involving both place and time has been made here.

minimal and did not live up to the hopes he had presumably pinned on a trip to a country where he had once been so celebrated. But this was no longer the rococo Paris of Louis XV. Even Boruwłaski noticed that everyone had been seized by political fever, and the new constitution was a topic of discussion not only among members of parliament but also aristocratic ladies. Concluding that he 'was swimming against the stream'[36] after not quite one year's stay in France, he decided to return to the British Isles.

In spring of 1791 he reached Guernsey, where he spent around two months, and returned to England for a short duration in June. But after a several-month trip on which he visited Hereford, Warwick, Coventry, then once again Birmingham, Derby, and Liverpool, among other locations, he headed for Ireland. This is when it seems that his wife left him. Indeed, it is hard to be surprised at her decision. The life the Boruwłaskis led must have been hard for a young woman burdened with small children: endless travel, a lack of basic conveniences, insufficient care for ailments related to her frequent pregnancies, constant uncertainty about the future, and lastly – perhaps even the most important factor – a sense of looking ridiculous, of being a laughing-stock. We should once again point out that Isalina was only 17 years old when she wed and had in a certain sense been forced into the marriage, having viewed it from the outset as humiliating to some extent. What must she have felt when it became her lot to perform together with her husband, to dance the 'Polish Cossack dance' with him in front of audiences, and allegedly even to carry him around in front of audiences in her arms?[37] Nothing is known about what happened to her for the next several decades, but it does seem that her separate life still remained full of colourful and exotic locales: she surfaces again in the historical record nearly half a century later in 1842, on the island of St Thomas in the Virgin Islands. There she lived with her daughter Fanny Georgiana, by then already a widow. The Virgin Islands was where Fanny's late husband, Patrick Kean from County Limerick, had had an estate. His Irish origins suggest that after splitting up with Boruwłaski, Isalina settled in Ireland together with her children and later accompanied her eldest daughter on her voyage to her husband's estate. Under

---

[36] *Memoirs* IV, p. 219.

[37] This is at least what Niemcewicz told Klementyna Hoffmanowa, *Przyjaciel Ludu* vol. 5, 1838, no. 16 / 20 Oct 1838.

Fanny's care she lived to the ripe old age of 90, dying in St Thomas in 1852. To the end of her life she continued using her married name – interestingly, with the correct feminine ending for a Polish surname: Boruwłaska.[38]

Joseph settled in Ireland for nearly six years, more or less from the end of 1792 to mid 1798, when he was chased away by the attempt made by French units to invade the island. The term 'settled' is an overstatement here, because these years were again essentially one ceaseless voyage for Boruwłaski. His predicament was not an easy one at that time. Alone, somewhat forgotten by his aristocratic protectors, left exclusively to his own devices, it was solely with his French servant Jean de Courcy, and after his death in 1795 with the Irishman Noad,[39] that he travelled throughout the island, calling at Dublin, Cork, Limerick, Galway, Sligo, Londonderry, Belfast, Armagh, Cavan, Kilkenny, Drogheda, and many other locations. All told, the places mentioned in the memoirs make for quite a detailed map of Ireland. He never stayed anywhere more than a few months. Everywhere he gave concerts, which he mentions in his memoirs, and everywhere he put himself on display for money, which he does not mention.

Despite his troublesome situation in life, Boruwłaski's recollections from Ireland are quite cheerful, and the problems he encountered along the way are treated more in jest, such as an innkeeper's coveting his purse, or the panic caused by the false rumour that General Louis-Lazare Hoche had landed at Bantry Bay in December 1796. He deemed the French general's act to be highly 'impolitic' or tactless, since he had deprived Boruwłaski of the profits he had expected to reap from a concert that ended up cancelled. This indeed shows the quintessence of Boruwłaski's stance towards politics. In any case, he was in Ireland during a time of intense political disputes, of clashes between Protestants and Catholics, of

---

[38]   This later portion of Izalina's life story, which I was previously unfamiliar with, comes courtesy of Mr Alain Duperon, who gave me copies of Georgiana Fanny Boruwłaska-Kean's letters to her children from 1842–1852 (mainly to her illegitimate daughter Julie Alphonsine), familiarised me with Maurice Devos's genealogical findings concerning the ancestors of the Favre family, which included Fanny Boruwłaska, and also provided me with information on the inscription borne on her tombstone at Montmartre cemetery in Paris. Fanny's letters are enchanting and her own life history is intriguing: suffice it to mention that she was born in London, spent a significant portion of her life on the Virgin Islands, only to end it in Paris. But that is a story for another book.

[39]   He only mentions Noad in the memoirs, but John S. Powell discovered a record of the death of a Jean de Courcy, '*valet du nain polonaise*', buried 24 April 1795, in the parish archives of the French church in Portarlington. J.S. Powell, op. cit., p. 5.

conspiracies, riots, unrest, and even a French attempt at invading the island, but almost nothing of this finds any refection in his memoirs. His only commentary about current events was a remark of regret that the times were not fortunate for him, because the public was generally focused more on politics than on entertainment.[40] Besides, it is hard to criticise him for this – in a certain sense Boruwłaski always remained 'outside' every society he lived in, and in Ireland he was moreover a foreigner with a poor grasp of the complexities of local politics. It was in his interest, and presumably in his character, to maintain good relations with anyone and everyone he came into contact with. In Ireland at that time, that probably required considerable diplomatic skill and an aptitude at delicately manoeuvring between representatives of various political forces. In any event, this was the only time Boruwłaski deemed it strategic to clearly underscore his lack of interest in politics. He did so quite prudently when talking to the commander of the British troops in Belfast, General George Nuget. He deftly insisted that the only politics he was interested in, and which he supported, was the 'politics of my tickets' – sold to his own concerts, of course.[41] From his perspective, the soldiers from the British garrison were just as good an audience as the 'good Irish people' in one town or another.[42]

It seems that Boruwłaski felt good in Ireland, and in any case he frequently stresses the kindness he encountered from people from diverse social circles. This portion of the memoirs highlights such diversity significantly more strongly. We encounter descriptions of meetings with Lord Ormond, his son Walter, and the abovementioned General Nuget, but also with representatives of essentially all the strata of Irish society, ranging from the proverbial 'poor peasants,' Quakers in Clonmell and Huguenot emigrants in Portarlington, to the Irish gentry and no less hospitable officers from the British garrisons. We learn that the author even visited a prison in Belfast at the invitation of the inmates, eager to see him first-hand, and received quite a warm reception there.[43] Here, too, is a whole gallery of colourful and amusing figures: there is a hypochondriac landlady in Portarlington, whom the author cured with a 'black powder' made of burnt bread, an apothecary in Athlone whose main skill 'consisted in the art of pickling

---

[40] *Memoirs* IV, p. 309.
[41] Ibidem, p. 304.
[42] Ibidem, p. 283.
[43] Ibidem, p. 287–289.

beef,' a Methodist preacher in Ballinasloe, angry at Boruwłaski for robbing him of listeners to preach to since they were more interested in seeing the small foreigner than in listening to a sermon, and a beautiful Mrs McLennel, the wife of a butcher in Cork, who prompted a language mistake made by Boruwłaski. When she promised to send him a 'marrow-bone' to his house, he misunderstood that she was referring to Mirabeau, and instead of a soup ingredient he was expecting a visit by the brother of the famous French politician.[44] Descriptions of people and events from the Irish stage of Boruwłaski's life are permeated with good-natured humour and mild irony, sometimes self-irony, which combined with the quite numerous anecdotes here make this one of the most cheerful fragments of the last edition of the memoirs.

The description of his further adventures is significantly less cheerful in tone. Steeped in the chaos of an uprising, facing an invasion by General Humbert, Ireland was no longer the hospitable asylum he was seeking – in the latter half of 1798 Boruwłaski left it in haste, to return to England after a short stay on the Isle of Man. The years 1799–1801 he probably spent in Newcastle;[45] later he came back to London. This was perhaps the worst period in his life. In principle things had not changed and he continued to travel, only this time around England, giving concerts, holding breakfasts, and exhibiting himself for money. He tried to increase his income somewhat by selling his memoirs, and from 1804 onward also by selling a sonata he composed 'for pianoforte or harpsichord.'[46] But he was already into his sixties, having spent 20 years in constant voyaging, and we can surmise that this lifestyle was becoming increasingly hard on him. Moreover, he was feeling an ever-greater need to secure his own future for his approaching old age. Around 1800, a hope arose for him to finally attain a certain financial stability when a collection of money was taken to set up an annuity fund for Boruwłaski. This was not the first such attempt. Boruwłaski mentions that the Duchess of Devonshire had had some sort of unrealised plans

---

[44]   Ibidem, p. 244.

[45]   It exists the announcements from the Newcastle press from 28 December 1799 (*Newcastle Courant* announcing his arrival) and from 27 June 1801 (*Newcastle Chronicle*).

[46]   *The Volunteer; New Sonata for the Pianoforte or Harpsichord*, composed by Count Joseph Boruwlaski, dedicated to the Hon. Mrs Buchanan, Edinburgh, (no date of publication). It was advertised in the press: *Glocester Journal*, 4 June 1804; *Bath Chronicle*, 24 Jan. 1805.

of this sort, and a subscription is known to have taken place in 1788[47] at the initiative of a mysterious Lady B. in Norwich,[48] with contributions coming from the Metcalfe sisters as well. But those efforts had not achieved the intended aim, probably at the fault of Boruwłaski himself, who too soon collected and spent the sum that had been gathered. He claimed that this had been done without his knowledge or consent by the French con-man Detreval.[49] This new initiative, in turn, did stand considerable chances of success, since it was promoted by the very influential Leonhard Smelt, a trusted friend of the king and his brother the Prince of Gloucester, who secured both of their support for the idea – this provided a financial boost as well as the prestige of royal involvement in the subscription. Unfortunately, even though a certain sum was amassed and entrusted to the Reverend Reynold Bouyer from Durham, the operation was never successfully finalised due to the sudden death of its organiser, Smelt, in September 1800. The subscription continued on,[50] but it does not seem to have yielded sufficient funds. In any case Boruwłaski was left still forced to exhibit himself in public. As late as mid 1805 he was still advertising in the *Morning Herald*, inviting London residents to attend a breakfast and promenade in his company in the Cumberland Gardens.[51] As he himself writes, his spirits sank so low that he even contemplated emigrating to America, to look for a means of living there.

It is hard to say how long this state of affairs continued. The present researcher has not managed to find any press announcements about Boruwłaski later than 1805, although we cannot conclude with certainty that there were none. He himself cautiously avoids giving any dates and he mixes up events somewhat or links together events separated in time – for instance the death of Mr Smelt (1800), the death of the Prince of Gloucester (1805), and the illness of George III (1810) are mentioned in the memoirs almost in parallel. It seems that 1805

---

[47] An announcement of the subscription appeared in the *Oxford Journal*, 6 Dec. 1788, and it is also mentioned by Boruwłaski in the last edition of his memoirs, p. 204 ff.

[48] Might this be the same person as the Mrs Buchanan to whom he dedicated his musical composition?

[49] *Memoirs* IV, p. 205 ff. Perhaps this was in fact the name of de Trouville, deformed years later?

[50] This was reported by the *Newcastle Chronicle*, 29 Aug. 1801.

[51] *Morning Herald*, 26 June 1805.

was when the final, at last fully successful attempt was made at collecting a sum of capital to ensure Boruwłaski an annual income sufficient for a decent life. This was done by his old friends the Metcalfe sisters, getting their own family involved as well as their title-bearing and wealthy acquaintances. Combined with the money gathered in the subscription organised by Smelt, this yielded a sum he could live on for the rest of his life, independently and relatively affluently.

Chapter 3

Józef Boruwłaski, Esq.

The money gathered by Joseph's friends and benefactors was invested in a lifetime annuity that ensured Boruwłaski an annual income of around 150 pounds.[1] The tale of the transaction itself was quite amusing, although perhaps not for everyone involved. The initial capital was given over to a wealthy merchant from Durham, who in exchange agreed to make the annuity payments to Boruwłaski for the remainder of his life. His purchase of the annuity was presumably motivated by the hope of earning considerable profits, given the advanced age of the beneficiary and the presumed likelihood of his death in the not-too-distant future. But Boruwłaski lived on and on. The merchant, though a decade and a half younger, was already ailing and elderly while Joseph remained in good health, and the amount of the annuity payments had long since exceeded the initial capital. Charles Mathews recalled a visit to Durham when Boruwłaski took him to visit the shop of a certain old man, with whom he exchanged some forced pleasantries. Boruwłaski reassured the man with great merriment that he was faring quite well and had felt 'never better.' Once out of earshot he could barely contain his laughter while explaining to Mathews that this had been the owner of his annuity, who was praying and praying for his death but 'Boruwlaski never die!'[2] Indeed, it seems that the obligation to make the annuity payments was even inherited by the hapless investor's children.

This level of annual income was not enough to enable Boruwłaski to settle permanently in London, where life was simply too expensive. He decided to settle in Durham, a town he had become familiar with several years previously during his travels, where he had struck up a warm friendship with Thomas

---

[1]   This is the sum (more precisely 138 pounds) that Boruwłaski states that he is earning in a letter to Emma George (26 Apr. 1826, Czartoryski Library, MS 2798), whereas the publisher 'Craftsman' estimated his income at 300 pounds in 1821 (8 Aug. 1821). In this case Boruwłaski himself seems to be a more credible source.

[2]   *Memoirs of Charles Mathews*, p. 223–225.

Ebdon, the organist at the cathedral. The precise date is unclear but he probably moved there around 1806.[3] At first it seems he lived with the Ebdon family. After Thomas's death in 1811, he moved to a small house reportedly designed by Bonomi, situated on the property at the address of 12 Old Bailey, not far from Prebend's Bridge, in the old part of Durham encircled by the Wear River.[4] There he lived to the end of his life, sustaining close bonds of friendship with Ebdon's daughters.

Boruwłaski cannot be said to have become a particularly wealthy man. The house in which he lived was extremely modest – small, dark, uncomfortable, and very humbly furnished.[5] But it seems that we can say that at the age of nearly 70 he finally attained what he had been striving for, if not for his whole life then at least for the last 30 years. He at long last became a financially independent man, able to settle down and become a fully-fledged member of a community, ceasing to be a public freak-show spectacle for the masses and a charming plaything of the high-and-mighty, but instead becoming simply Mr Boruwłaski, a pleasant, witty, and small gentleman. Recollections of him from this period underscore greatly how jovial a person he was, referring both to his cheerfulness, which was always a point of admiration, and his sense of humour – sometimes he was even described as a wit and jokester.[6] He quickly became

---

[3]   This would be confirmed by the date of his acceptance into the local Masonic lodge, in 1806 (information from Mrs Margot Johnson, regional historian of Durham and its vicinities). Cf. also R.F. Gould, 'Freemasonry in Cheshire', *Ars Quatuor Coronatorum*, 15, 1902, pp. 41–45.

[4]   'He lived in a tiny little Greek-temple-like house which, built by Mr Bonomi the architect, stood by the river very near Prebend's Bridge. It was quite out of place where it was, but I was almost sorry to see that it had gone when, being on a visit Durham, I took my children to see it.' *Account of her early life by Margaret Hunt*, in *A Raine Miscellany*, ed. by Angela Marsden, The publications of the Surtees Society, vol. 200, 1991, p. 125.

[5]   This judging by the *Catalogue of Furniture, Books and other Effects of the Late Celebrated Polish Dwarf Count Boruwlaski, to be sold by auction … the 29th Day of November 1838*. All of his personal articles, including a sizeable library, were appraised at less than 100 pounds.

[6]   'The Count was an excellent wit and humourist', *The Times* 13 Sept. 1837; 'His responses were lively and witty, and his conversation highly engaging', letter from Mr Scheilds of Durham to Krystyn Lach Szyrma, 27 Sept. 1837, cited from the Polish translation published in *Przyjaciel Ludu*, vol. 5, Leszno, 1838, p. 126.

popular in the town and its environs.[7] He revived his old friendships among the acting community – his closest associate in Durham was Stephen Kemble, until the latter's death in 1822.[8] Their frequent walks together must have offered quite an amusing sight, since Kemble was a man of such sizeable build that he could play Falstaff without any special preparations. Boruwłaski also made many new acquaintances. His entry into local society was presumably facilitated by his Masonic membership – as early as in 1806 he had became an honorary member of the local organisation (Granby Lodge), to which Kemble likewise belonged. On the other hand, he was not a very active member and only attended three lodge meetings.[9] His intelligence, humour, and extraordinary cheerful character won him many friends among the local gentry, which listened with fascination to the stories of his travels and the years of his youth spent in the courts of the grand monarchs. Through his friend Ebdon, and then through Ebdon's nephew Stephen (the canon of the Cathedral in Durham), he was involved in the social life of the college of canons, making many acquaintances among the local clergy – numerous names of clergymen are mentioned in the last edition of his memoirs and also appear among its subscribers. Boruwłaski was familiar with the Reverend Adam Clarke, a well-known publisher and biblical scholar, and who hosted him at his home.[10] He became friends with James Raine, one of the most outstanding representatives of Durham's intellectual elite, the rector of St Mary-the-Less and a founder of the University of Durham, a historian and antiquarian. These were lively and close contacts. Boruwłaski was also a frequent guest at Raine's home, and even took part in family events, such as his son's christening. This visit was recalled by the rector's daughter, then (in the early 1830s) a small child, who wrote years later about how she had been taken aback by his unusual appearance and kept asking: 'Man? Boy?'[11] These acquaintances, lasting and clearly a source of satisfaction for both sides, seem to confirm that Boruwłaski not only knew how to entertain but also how to take part in more

---

[7] *The Life and Love Letters of a Dwarf*, p. 153, publisher's notes; T. Heron, op. cit., p. 17.

[8] *A Series*, p. 330; *Notes and Queries* August 1857, p. 158, the account of James Raine.

[9] Information from Margot Johnson; R.F. Gould, op. cit., p. 41 ff.; *Memoirs* IV, p. 232.

[10] *Notes and Queries*, May 1856, p. 358.

[11] *Account of her early life by Margaret Hunt*, in *A Raine Miscellany*, ed. by A. Marsden, The publications of the Surtees Society, vol. 200, 1991.

serious discussions about cultural or scientific matters. There is one more piece of evidence pointing in this direction: his library. The catalogue drawn up for an auction after his death lists precisely what it contained. Considering its owner's limited resources, this was a sizeable collection numbering around 200 volumes, and it fully confirmed the favourable opinions about Boruwłaski's intelligence. Aside from encyclopaedic and dictionary publications (Boyer's *Dictionnaire*, *Penny Cyclopaedia*), old periodicals (*Spectator*), and current ones (*London Magazine*, *Town and Country Magazine*), they included many historical treatises (including an English history of Poland) and classics – authors of antiquity (Plutarch and Aesop) and works by Shakespeare, Molière, Milton. The volumes of belles-lettres were dominated by British Enlightenment authors in both prose (Swift, Goldsmith) and poetry (Pope, Young, Thompson).[12] In general the collection evidenced a clear predominance of volumes in English, indicating that Boruwłaski read freely in the language. This was the library of a man of quite conservative tastes: it effectively does not contain any nineteenth-century literature, and one could even conclude that the collection had been put together long before its owner had come to live in Durham and was no longer expanded after that. At the same time it was the collection of a refined man with broad interests (including books on natural history and travel). Perhaps once he settled down for good, Boruwłaski no longer felt any need to accumulate books, instead tapping into the local library and the collections of his friends.

We have information about few events from the 30-year period of Boruwłaski's life in Durham. But on the other hand, this was most likely not a time very full of dramatic incidents. We might conclude, following his contemporary commentators, that he resided there peacefully, 'universally respected by all classes.'[13] Apart from his lively social life, he was fond of tending his garden and is also said to have dabbled in experimenting with alchemy, allegedly in the hope of finding the philosopher's stone – these rumours indeed seem to find some confirmation in the chemical equipment that ended up listed among the articles of his estate: small copper and bronze scales, including a special scale for gold, and also works by Paracelsus and Galen.[14] As long as his health permitted, every

---

[12]   *Catalogue of Furniture* (no date of publication).

[13]   *Biographia Curiosa*, p. 79.

[14]   Scheilds to Krystyn Lach Szyrma, 27 Sep. 1837, op. cit., p. 126; *Catalogue of Furniture* (no date of publication).

year he travelled to London to stay for a few weeks with the Mathews family, for whom he became something like a member of the household, and from there he would be invited to spend long visits with his old friends the Metcalfe sisters.

Around 1816 he set about drawing up another version of his memoirs, this time in English. He was helped in this task by the writer William Burdon. The latter must have provided no small assistance indeed, considering Boruwłaski's 'prettily broken English,' as it was then described. Although he spoke English freely, he never really learned to speak it grammatically and pronounced it with a very distinct accent. He wrote of himself: 'I am slow writer in English.'[15] The memoirs were published in 1820 and were dedicated to King George IV. Their appearance thus served as an opportunity to visit the monarch – undoubtedly the most important event from this period of Boruwłaski's life. Through the efforts of Charles Mathews and the mediation of Lord Conyngham, a royal audience was successfully arranged for him in July 1821, just before the King's ceremonious coronation. The ruler received Boruwłaski in his private apartments at Carlton House, treating him as an old friend and recalling their acquaintance back when he was still Prince of Wales. Their conversation was in French, the King was enchanted with his guest, and even confided to Mathews that Boruwłaski was for him a paragon of good behaviour and elegance, and at the same time the most refined and charming individual he knew. Although he inquired about whether Boruwłaski might need support, he did so very delicately, asking Mathews on the side so as not to offend the little Pole. He not only treated him as a gentleman but also addressed him very warmly, among other things offering him a chance to view his coronation robes. While showing them to Boruwłaski he advised him against attending the coronation itself, as such a large crowd might be dangerous for him. It is easy to guess that Boruwłaski was simply elated. Mathews, to whom we owe the description of this visit, wrote that after returning home his friend (then 84 years old) 'danced and pirouetted' out of joy.[16]

Mathews reports that a certain 'vivacity of temperament' was one of Boruwłaski's characteristic traits; other witnesses state that at the age of 80 he

---

[15]   J. Boruwłaski to Emma George, 27 May 1826, Czartoryski Library 2798.
[16]   *Memoirs of Charles Mathews*, p. 217–230.

exuded simply boyish behaviour and merriment.[17] In part this was probably because he was a child of an epoch then long past, when people did not shrink from showing emotions, but it was probably to a greater degree a result of Boruwłaski's own personality. Mathews's account of Boruwłaski is all the more valuable in that they knew one another closely for a long time – they first met in Norwich in 1788 and encountered one another regularly starting in 1805.[18] To Mathews and his wife, Boruwłaski was a friend, not a freak of nature. In truth Charles does poke fun at his behaviour somewhat, above all the way he spoke English, but at the same time he repeatedly stresses Boruwłaski's intelligence, common sense, and gaiety, recognising him as a fascinating personality and a charming comrade.[19] An interesting difference can be sensed between Mathews's recollections and the account of Peter Patmore, who got to know Boruwłaski at the Mathews home. For Patmore, Boruwłaski's physique is still important. At least at the time they met, he regarded Boruwłaski as 'one of those miracles of mechanism about which we read' and scrupulously notes details of his appearance and behaviour.[20] But it seems that Patmore, too, ended up succumbing to Joseph's personal charm, since his writings move from rapture at his 'child-like innocence' to admiration for his brilliant intellect and splendid skill at engaging in interesting discussion, and finally to fascination at what he called Boruwłaski's 'little microcosm of his own mind and character.'[21] Indeed, even though Patmore's recollections of Joseph may initially seem very similar to opinions voiced about Joujou 60 years earlier, back at the outset of his career, one can sense a certain subtle yet significant shift in tone, towards a perspective that is all the more distinct in Mathews's writings. In the years of his youth Boruwłaski's height was always at the forefront, and his intelligence was more of a pleasant and to a certain degree even surprising addition, something that was essentially not expected from someone of his physique. But in later accounts, admiration for the virtues of Boruwłaski's intellect and character is something independent of the

---

[17] Account of Peter R. Pattmore, included in *Memoirs of Charles Mathews*, p. 231.

[18] *Memoirs* IV, p. 204; Mathews gives no date for their first meeting.

[19] *Memoirs of Charles Matthews* p. 213.

[20] As R.H. Heatley described it: 'as if he were an animated musical toy,' *The Life and Love Letters*, p. 154.

[21] *Memoirs of Charles Mathews*, p. 231.

interest attracted by his abnormal height. For those who knew him well, like Mathews, the issue of his appearance simply recedes into the background, and although superficial acquaintances like Patmore may have been enraptured with his dainty build, even they ended up impressed by his prowess of mind. And this feeling was no longer expressed the way it had been by the Count de Tressan, as a sense of astonishment that Boruwłaski was 'so small, yet so intelligent,' but rather as simple admiration for his intellect and character in their own right, irrespective of his intriguing smallness. This was perhaps Boruwłaski's greatest success, one that attests to both the change in his situation and to the charm of his personality.

Boruwłaski thus finally managed to free himself from the role that life had imposed upon him: the internationally acclaimed dwarf was at long last replaced by Joseph Boruwłaski Esquire. This does not mean that his 'miracle of nature' guise was entirely forgotten, but it receded into the background – or perhaps more accurately we should say that a kind of separation of roles occurred, one being the real Mr Boruwłaski, popular and well-liked by his friends and acquaintances, the other being a lingering legend. Although he ceased to exhibit himself in public, the public memory of him nevertheless persisted. No publication surveying various miracles and wonders of nature could fail to mention him: *The New Wonderful Museum* from 1804 and *Biografia Curiosa* and *Wonderful Characters*, both from 1822, devoted much attention to 'the most astonishing dwarf' Boruwłaski, published portraits of him, and cited or summarised fragments of his memoirs. From time to time his name was recalled in press reports, which alongside his numerous admirable traits now began to mention his very advanced age. For example, in 1821 the *Craftsman* reported: 'The extraordinary and accomplished Polish dwarf, Count Bouwlaski [!] is still living and is now in the 82 year of his age.'[22] However, this was a legend that already functioned essentially without the involvement of its object. For the residents of Durham, Boruwłaski may perhaps have been something of a point of pride (as is attested by the mention of him and his home in Metcalf Ross's

---

[22] *Craftsman*, 3 Aug. 1821.

unique description of the town, dated 1834),[23] but he was above all a pleasant neighbour.

The difference in how he was perceived is well illustrated by fragments of two recollections written after his death, the first carried in the obituaries section of the *Times* (cited from the *Newcastle Chronicle*) began: 'The Polish Dwarf Count Boruwlaski. His person, though of diminutive formation, was of the completest symmetry, his height being about 36 inches,' then continued on to briefly recap his life in Britain up until he settled in Durham and to mention the virtues of his intellect and character.[24] The second death notice, published in the *The Durham Advertiser*, states: 'At his residence near Prebend's Bridge on Tuesday last [died] in the 99th year of his age Count Joseph Boruwlaski, a native of the province of Pokucia in the Polish Russia. The extraordinary small stature, great age and lively genious of this amiable little gentleman, entitled him to be ranked as one of the most singular productions of nature; while his long residence in this city and cheerful demeanour, both greatly endeared him to a numerous circle of friends and acquaintants, by whom his loss will be long and sincerely regretted.'[25] These would seem to be quite similar announcements, yet note how very different they really are: one speaks of a Polish dwarf whose height had been so important that it is cited almost at the very outset, the other speaks of a Polish count whose short size had been distinctive, but no more so than his longevity or lively intellect, and who had simply been a neighbour and friend.

Boruwłaski very much prized this image of his as an autonomous gentleman. He takes great satisfaction in noting in his memoirs that he did not accept an offer of financial assistance from Mr Burdon, because he no longer needed such assistance.[26] We can understand his pride: this seems to have been the very first

---

[23]　'From the Palace Green is an avenue leading to the public walks, called "The Banks" [...] Immediately contiguous to the New Bridge [Prebend's Bridge] stands a neat cottage, the miniature representation of a Grecian temple, in which resides the celebrated Polish dwarf count Joseph Boruwlaski.' 'In reality, the ease and politeness of his manners and address please no less than the diminutive, yet elegant proportions of his figure, astonish those who visit him,' M. Ross, *A Historical and Descriptive View of the City of Durham*, Newcastle upon Tyne, 1834, p. 219–220 – this publication was produced in just two copies, and also included a pasted-in autograph of Boruwłaski.

[24]　*The Times*, 13 Sept. 1837; a similar text in *Watchman* 27 Sept. 1837.

[25]　*The Durham Advertiser*, 8 Sept. 1837.

[26]　*Memoirs* IV, p. 374.

time in his life he was able to turn such a hand-out down. How important this was for him is shown by how greatly anxious he became prior to his audience with George IV, when he confided to his friend his great angst that the King might offer him money. He was afraid that the monarch, aware of his life story, might conclude that he was not a man of honour and was simply there to seek support. Boruwłaski felt that such a gift would have hurt his pride and humiliated him forever; he was allegedly even close to tears at the very thought.[27] Fortunately the ruler respected his guest's honour and offered him a costly watch as a memento.

Interestingly, even though Boruwłaski had not been in Poland for several decades and essentially did not maintain any contacts with his native land, it remained a standing element of his image that he was a 'Polish nobleman.' This he stressed in his memoirs, even adding in the last edition several bits of information describing various attractions in the country, such as the Wieliczka Salt Mine, Lake Żórawno, and so on. He must have also stressed this in his conversations, since nearly every recollection of him mentions his link to Poland. That seems quite natural – after all, his objective through his entire life was to verify his status as the Imć Pan Boruwłaski – Honourable Joseph Boruwłaski, a member of the Polish nobility.

Boruwłaski lived out his final years in Durham under the care of Elizabeth and Mary Ebdon. He enjoyed considerable interest and would pose for painters and sculptors. We might say that he became a permanent fixture in the city's panorama, turning up in Durham landscapes painted by local artists.[28] From time to time an acquaintance from the old days would re-establish contact with him, such as Catherine Hutton, who approached him in 1833 asking for an autograph for her collection, or the nephew of his Edinburgh acquaintance Neil Fergusson, who visited him in 1836.[29] Reports stressed how he remained very mentally fit to the very end of his days. He died on 5 September 1837 at the ripe old age of 98 and was buried in Durham Cathedral. To this day his grave is marked by a stone bearing the letters 'J.B.' A plaque commemorating him was also installed in St Mary-the-Less church. But he himself penned his own

---

27   *Memoirs of Charles Mathews*, p. 221.

28   He can be seen in paintings by Joseph Bouet (showing the entrance gate of the old prison in Durham) and James Terry (a view of the northern facade of the cathedral), both dating from the early 1820s.

29   C. Hutton, op. cit., p. 249; *A series*, p. 330.

most apt epitaph, when he sent Catherine Hutton this verse as his autograph: 'Poland was my cradle,/England is my nest;/Durham is my quiet place,/Where my bones shall rest.'[30]

---

[30]   C. Hutton, op. cit., p. 249.

Chapter 4

Boruwłaski's Two Guises

Many times while recounting Boruwłaski's life here we have made specific references to his memoirs, both the earlier and the later versions, above all treating them as a source of more or less reliable information. However, this publication – or rather these publications – certainly deserve more cautious and more careful attention, especially because they have not attracted much interest specifically as a work of literature. It seems that both English- and Polish-speaking researchers have adopted the opinion expressed by the author of the preface to the second edition: 'The facts pointed out in this history are by no means important: they are in no wise connected with the great events of Europe, which so strongly impress all nations; they bear a proportion to the object described; they are in a manner correspondent to his size.'[1] Indeed, history with a capital 'H' is absent from the memoirs. As we have already noted, the author fails to notice the ongoing partitions of Poland, the French Revolution nearly escapes his attention, and he remains focused on himself, on his own predicament and emotions, on the events he took part in first-hand. But is that sufficient reason to overlook what the content of his memoirs can tell us about the times in which he lived? There are indeed some intriguing surprises awaiting scholars willing to invest the time and effort. One crucial point that has to date most evidently escaped readers' attention is that there exist two significant versions of the memoirs, differing so much from each other that one might be tempted to conclude that they report the lives of two different people. Boruwłaski thus presents himself to us in two completely different guises, worthy of careful analysis and comparison.

But first, we need to bring a bit more clarity to the issue of the successive editions of these memoirs, since considerable chaos has prevailed in this regard. This is especially true for Polish analyses and bibliographies, although scholarly work in English has also failed to settle these issues clearly and conclusively. The

---

[1] *Memoirs* II, introduction, p. xxx ff.

very first, bilingual edition was published in 1788.[2] Here the original French text was translated into English by Jean Thomas Hérissant Des Carrières, and this is definitely the best of all English translations of the memoirs. A German translation was published in Leipzig in 1790,[3] and two more editions, this time separately in French and English, appeared in Birmingham in 1792.[4] The memoirs were published two more times during the author's lifetime – a third English edition, being a reprint (perhaps an unauthorised one?) of the 1792 English edition, came out in 1801,[5] and then another version, the fourth and final edition published while Boruwłaski was still alive, appeared in 1820.[6] We have repeatedly noted above how this last 1820 edition differed in numerous aspects from the previous ones, but a closer look reveals such differences to be so fundamental that the 1820 version should essentially be considered a different book altogether. The memoir's twentieth-century publisher expressed regret in his notes that the author's 'individuality' gets completely lost in the fourth and final version, pinning the blame for this firmly on the translator.[7] But as we will discuss below, perhaps this lost personality was not just Mr Burdon's fault.

However, we need to start our examination by considering the first edition of the memoirs, not only on chronological grounds but also because it represents the author's greatest literary achievement. That is somewhat paradoxical, given

---

2   *Mémoires du célébre nain Joseph Boruwlaski gentilhomme polonois* ... écrits par lui meme en français et traduit en anglais par des Carrières, London, 1788.

3   *Leben des bekannten Zwerges Joseph Boruwlaski, eines polnischen Edelmans.* Aus dem Englischen [übersetst C.A. Wichmann], Leipzig, 1790.

4   *Mémoires du célébre nain Joseph Boruwlaski gentilhomme polonois* ... écrits par lui meme, revus, corrigés et augmentés, Birmingham: J. Thompson, 1792; *A Second Edition of the Memoirs of the Celebrated Dwarf Joseph Boruwlaski, a Polish Gentleman*, carefully revised and corrected, and translated from the French by Mr S. Freeman, Birmingham: J. Thompson, 1792 (in reality this was a corrected version, in some places quite heavily corrected, of Carrières's translation, extended to include closing fragments). Referred herein to as '*Memoirs* II.'

5   *Memoirs of the Celebrated Dwarf Joseph Boruwlaski, a Polish Gentleman*, translated from the original French ... and carefully revised and corrected, Kelso: James Ballantyne, 1801.

6   *Memoirs of Count Boruwlaski: containing a sketch of his travels, with an account at the different courts of Europe written by himself*, corrected by Mr Burdon, Durham: F. Humble, 1820. Referred herein to as '*Memoirs* IV.'

7   '[It] was "corrected" by Mr Burdon with so free a hand that the individuality of the author is completely lost,' *The Life and Love letters*, p. xiv.

that this first edition definitely encompasses less content than the final edition. In essence, when presenting his travels for the first time in 1788, Boruwłaski highlighted two things: his salon talents and his oddity. The Europe he takes us wandering through was one of enlightened courts and salons. This is nothing surprising in that he knew no other Europe. Boruwłaski himself, his way of looking at the world, was shaped by the culture of the salons, in a certain sense he was an ideal product of those salons. Even the most ardent frequenters of high-society gatherings still spent at least some part of their lives outside the salons: they took part in political, scholarly, economic life, they had family ties and personal contacts extending into the outside world. For Boruwłaski the salon was essentially the only world he knew and understood. As we have already noted, more or less from the fifteenth to the 40th year of his life, he lived practically in complete isolation from the surrounding realities. The salon-within-a-salon created for him by the Countess Humiecka may serve as a kind of symbol of his situation. The boundaries of the salon were at least up to a certain moment the outer limits of his world, and he described his successes in the terms of that world. We might say that in general he perceived nothing beyond it. His reflections about his trip through Holland are telling in this regard: first he gives a perfunctory report of his admiration at the Dutch countryside, then states: 'It would be repeating what has been said a thousand times, if I undertook to describe it; I will then confine myself to say, that when we arrived at the Hague, this astonishing village, which may vie with cities of the first rank, the Countess Humiecka was received in the most affable and polite manner by his Highness the Prince Stadtholder and his family, who did their utmost to make her stay agreeable. We, however, made but few acquaintances there.' In a certain sense this short passage captures the very essence of the memoirs. The travellers were 'received in the most affable and polite manner' at the royal courts, they made a sensation in the salons. 'On our return to Paris, the curiosity I excited drew many visitors to my protectress; and in less than a week, every person of high rank at court, every person of fashion in town waited upon her. I could not help, indeed, being infinitely flattered by that kind of enthusiasm and the numberless civilities I was honoured with.' Boruwłaski presents himself to readers as the perfect man-of-the-world, or perhaps more accurately as the perfect plaything for polite society. He does seem to have been excellently aware of his own predicament:

'Those, however, would be much mistaken, who should imagine that, seduced by the repeated kindnesses bestowed on me [...] I could always be unconscious of being, upon the whole, only looked upon by others as a doll, a little more perfect, it is true, and better organised that they commonly are, but however only as an animated toy.'

This leads us to the second dominant theme of the first edition of the memoirs: the physical deformity of their author. Our analysis of the memoirs should not lose sight of the author's overarching objective: to earn as much money as possible from their publication and thus improve his family's situation. Boruwłaski himself made no secret of that fact, as is confirmed by the broad subscription efforts and by the advertising campaign carried out in February 1787.[8] As the newspaper reports stated, these memoirs were intended to satisfy the public curiosity about 'the particulars of his travels, no less interesting than the account of his birth and person.'[9] As is understandable in this situation, both the subscription announcements and the lengthy descriptions of the memoirs especially showcased the author's physical oddity – obviously meant to be the book's main selling point.

In a certain sense, although the memoirs contain few descriptions of the community within which Boruwłaski functioned, we can still deduce quite a bit about it. The Europe of the enlightened salons and courts, seen through the eyes of Gulliver in the land of the giants, reveals to us a face that we are not very familiar with, one which its representatives would probably not have been very proud of. We should here remember that the memoirs were intended for readers from these very circles, and the author tried to highlight anything and everything that might interest them. Hence it is important not only what he describes, but also why he decided to describe a certain event. As we can deduce from the memoirs, his experience with the enlightened elite had taught Boruwłaski that he was interesting to them mainly in view of his oddity. He realised full well that both his aristocratic subscribers and individuals purchasing the book after visiting his home were not interested in his story per se, but just wanted to read as much as possible about his deformity. Hence, while he repeatedly insisted

---

[8]   Subscription announcements in the *Morning Post*, 13 Feb. 1787, 24 Apr. 1787; a review encouraging readers to buy the book in the *Morning Herald*, 29 May 1788; a sizeable summary in the *Bath Chronicle*, 7 Aug. 1788.

[9]   *Morning Post*, 24 Apr. 1787.

in the memoirs that his perception of the world and his sensibilities were no different from other people's, at the same time he specifically showcased those events from his life that were meant to underscore his peculiarity and oddity. The book's title alone stressed that readers would learn about the sensational life of the 'celebrated dwarf', whereas the text included detailed accounts of his brawl with Stanisław Leszczyński's dwarf Nicolas Ferry (Bébé) when our hero nearly ended up perishing in the fireplace, about how Count Ogiński had him served up to guests at a table inside an urn for amusement, about how people openly debated the sexual capabilities of dwarfs in his presence, and so on. Moreover, the author included these incidents as if against his own emotions, seeing those situations as humiliating. This can be said for many of the scenes described in the first edition of the memoirs – especially since there is no reason to doubt the author's own sensitivities, something he repeatedly brings up. In a certain sense, the literary form of this first edition of the memoirs is the product of a clash between the author's own sensitivities and the necessity he faced, stemming from purely mercantile motives, of making a show out of his deformity. And so, if we were to try to name a literary precursor, we would have to look not among the works of the great memoirists painting grand panoramas of their epochs, such as St Simon, but instead look to a completely different genre, one whose master was Jean-Jacques Rousseau. Boruwłaski's recollections sit well within the 'confessions' genre, popular at that time. It is worth noting that even the world of the courts and salons is described quite superficially in his memoirs, serving as a kind of background to his own introspective thoughts and feelings. This makes it even less surprising that the book fails to cover major political events or provide descriptions of the countries he visits. Even if the author had taken an interest in such things, there would not have been any place for them.

The chosen convention did, on the other hand, afford ample room for introspective analyses of his psychological states, meticulous descriptions of the author's feelings, including the indignities he suffered on account of his diminutive size. Boruwłaski spared his readers none of this. Suffice it to recall his description of his emergence into adult life and his first romance, which ended in painful disappointment and humiliation. Similarly, his 'romance' with Isalina is presented with simply astonishing frankness. The remainder of the story, recounting the fate of the Boruwłaskis wandering through Europe and then through Britain, is as much a description of events (and a list of donations received) as it is a catalogue of the author's states of mind – from euphoria at achieving matrimonial success to painful concern for his own fate and that of his burgeoning family, from pride at his contacts with the powerful elite to humiliation at the need to put himself on public display. Facts and events are evaluated from this subjective perspective. It seems that the choice of specifically this convention for the memoirs, a conscious choice we can assume, was an apt decision and the first edition can be declared a success for Boruwłaski as a writer.

But he himself does not seem to have been satisfied. That is already suggested by the alterations that were made to the second edition, and is clearly confirmed by the last edition. Because Boruwłaski, it seems, judged his own recollections in personal terms, not literary ones. We can conclude that he had included certain scenes in the first edition as a way to amuse the masses, much as he put his own body on display. Already in the second edition, he decided that some of the details would better be left unsaid. The key decision here was the already-mentioned removal of nearly all of his correspondence with Isalina – leaving just Joujou's final two letters from 20 and 27 November. This change distinctly alters the force of that portion of the memoirs – the reader learns nothing about the young lady's misgivings or even aversion to the idea, instead taking away the impression that their affections were mutual and outside factors alone stood in the way. That undoubtedly puts the author in better light, but it also had a decidedly negative impact on the literary value of the memoirs, deprived of their best fragment. But as we have already said, Boruwłaski was not guided here by aesthetic considerations. That is shown by other, small corrections the author introduces in the course of the narration. There are not yet many of them in this edition, but those that are there are quite telling. A good example is the story of how Anna Humiecka took him under her patronage. In the first edition, the Countess Tarnowska's motive for giving up the small Joujou was the fear that living with a dwarf in her midst while pregnant might possibly end up causing her to give birth to a deformed child. In the second edition, this was replaced by a sentimental tale about how Humiecka had persuaded Tarnowska that maternal love for the child she was then carrying would not permit her to devote enough attention to Boruwłaski, and that she herself would care for him more tenderly.[10] Another, even more telling alteration was made to just a single sentence in the account about the papal nuncio's objection to the notion of his marriage. In the first edition it reads: 'The Pope's Nuncio wanted to prevent it, as being disproportionate.' In the second it becomes: 'The Pope's Nuncio wanted to prevent it, by a ridiculous pretext.'[11] While this might not seem like a great difference, it certainly was one from the author's perspective. But still, these alterations did not yet affect the overall form of the memoirs and the second issue, like the first, maintains the same very personal and introspective tone.

The real watershed would not come until the fourth and last edition of the memoirs. Even an external glance at the 1820 edition suggests it is fundamentally different: this book expanded upon the author's life story to such a great extent that the text runs more than twice as long as previous versions, coming in at 391 pages, whereas the 1792 edition contained only 132 pages of approximately similar format. Boruwłaski's corrections and supplementations to the second edition were generally small and mostly pertained to events that had occurred since the last printing. But the additions to the 1820 edition include not only events that had occurred since 1792, but also, more surprisingly, numerous new travels and adventures in the preceding period, already covered in depth in the first edition. Aside from smaller additions interspersed in various places of the text, three new chapters appear in between his description of his arrival to Austria and his departure for the German principalities, portraying voyages which Boruwłaski obviously never actually took – at the very least because, as we have already written, he simply did not have the time for that to be possible. He must have drawn his descriptions of those exotic places he allegedly visited from the accounts of other travellers.

However, it is not these easy-to-notice additions that make it so worthwhile to analyse latter edition closely, carefully comparing it to the previous ones, especially the first. Subtler changes are even more important: the quiet omission of certain episodes, their replacement with others. Certain shifts of emphasis, we might say, that change the way the author is presented and alter the tone of his writing. This self-projected identity, or rather identities, are what make Boruwłaski's memoirs particularly interesting. The magnitude of the difference

---

[10]   *Memoirs* II, p. 9.
[11]   *Memoirs* II, p. 75.

is already suggested by the titles of the books: all the previous editions have the description 'celebrated dwarf' in their titles (*célèbre nain, bekannte Zwerg*), whereas the 1820 edition is offered to readers simply as the *Memoirs of Count Boruwlaski*, without so much as hinting at the author's abnormal size. The choice of frontispiece illustration is also indicative: no longer is there a tiny father playing with a child larger than him, held in its mother's arms (like in the first edition), nor an elegant dwarf carrying an epée (like in the second edition). The engraving by Joseph Bouet chosen in 1820 shows Boruwłaski in a close-up view, so that it would be hard to say anything about his size if it were not for the contour outline of his conversation-partner's silhouette. Unlike the previous images, this portrait does not in any way give the impression of a toy or an astonishing phenomenon of nature, it is simply a faithful representation of the author's appearance. These two differences, of title and opening illustration, encapsulate the whole issue: the earlier editions were the memoirs of a dwarf who was at the same time a Polish nobleman, whereas the last edition retraces the adventures of a Polish count who just happened to have received from nature an extraordinarily small stature. The question arises of whether this all amounts to vacuous word-play describing one and the same thing. But it seems that it was not: the author himself does seem to have gone to considerable effort to achieve precisely this effect.

He changed not only the title of the book, but its content and form as well. Above all, the scenes that the author deemed to have impinged upon his dignity disappeared – there is no recounting of the dinner at Ogiński's, his scuffle with Leszczyński's dwarf, or blatant discussion of his sexual capacity, no description of his meeting with a giant, no mention of the romantic affairs of his youth, the story of his feelings for Isalina, or details of his family life. This last omission was at least in part motivated by the fact that his marriage had broken apart many years previously and the author was most likely not fond of recalling it. The other events were closely related to the author's abnormality, which in this draft of the memoirs receded into the background or at least is no longer the 'main attraction' as it was in the previous editions. This difference was undoubtedly caused by the change in the author's situation, chiefly his financial stabilisation. Although he was once again hoping to earn some sort of income from the memoirs, he no longer had to try to attract readership at all costs – and definitely not at the price of humiliation or making a laughingstock of himself. To the extent of his ability, Boruwłaski also avoids recalling that he was ever forced to exhibit himself for money, writing mainly about his concerts as if they were the performances of an ordinary travelling virtuoso. There is also much less complaining in this edition about being treated like a child. We can say that unlike the previous editions, he no longer reassures readers about his similarity to other people as much as he simply demonstrates that similarity by means of the stories he relates. The added descriptions of events, in which his adventures and impressions do not differ from those of other voyagers, seem to serve this purpose. Indeed, not just the content of the narration, but also its tone has changed – this is not a frank confession but an event-reporting tale, and the author has learned to observe events and his own person with a sense of detachment. Boruwłaski gives readers a clear signpost for how they should treat his memoirs. To his description of the sensation he caused in Paris upon arriving there with Humiecka, he added a telling remark: 'So that I became like Gulliver with his master the farmer.'[12] This one sentence alters in a distinctive way the author's perspective and stance towards the surrounding world. Here we have not the personal confessions of a man wronged by nature, but the recollections of a traveller of small size roaming the world of big people not without amusing mishaps. Elsewhere Boruwłaski presents himself as 'a man that had to make my way round the world, to support my existence, and study the human mind.'[13] Thus it is not surprising that little remains in the fourth and final edition of the previous introspection and analysis of Boruwłaski's own feelings. The author instead tries to portray himself more as a careful observer armed with a witty and at times even brilliant sense of humour. He even musters up a sense of self-irony, something that was practically absent from the previous editions. He does not even shy away from describing amusing situations he found himself in: such as an adventure involving a mastiff sleeping under his bed, when Boruwłaski ended up landing in a nearby washtub and was convinced he was experiencing an earthquake – much to the amusement of his chance acquaintances at the inn.[14] There are more such anecdotes, but although they are undoubtedly amusing they are not humiliating, they do not injure the

---

[12] *Memoirs* IV, p. 35.
[13] *Memoirs* IV, p. 285, cf. a similar remark on p. 378.
[14] *Memoirs* IV, p. 161–164.

author's personal dignity. Moreover, they are generally unrelated to his height and to all extents and purposes they could have happened to anyone else.

When evaluating the last edition of the memoirs, we can observe a kind of feedback in action: changes in content triggered changes in form, which in turn triggered further changes in the book's content. Once the author abandoned his former personal tone of frank confession, cast off his former introspection and subjective evaluation of events from a very individual perspective, and left out the issues that were touchier for him, what was left over from the first version of the memoirs was just a skeleton, a text too meagre to spark much interest. Hence the need to add new material, to develop new narrative threads, to replace the omitted anecdotes with new ones. And that is precisely what the author did. Perhaps this decision was in some way guided by the timing of when he was preparing this last version for publication. In the nineteenth century, sentimental tenderness and 'confessions' so frank as to be painful, nearly exhibitionist, had long since gone out of fashion and the author may have feared that such a book would not have found too many readers. The world of the enlightened salons, which had long ceased to exist, also presumably would not have attracted much interest. But travel stories certainly still enjoyed unabating popularity, hence the choice of this particular genre as a model. And so, Boruwłaski takes readers from one end of Europe to the other and on excursions to Asia and Africa, regales them with new tales, and recounts to them his own alleged polemics with Dr Johnson and his nearly philosophical deliberations about virtue and the role of public opinion.

The question still remains of what role was actually played by William Burdon, named as having 'corrected' the fourth edition of the memoirs – which given Boruwłaski's poor knowledge of English must have meant that he simply translated them. But unlike for previous editions we do not possess any original French text, and indeed such a version most likely never existed, with the book instead being drafted directly in English by two men at the same time – the author and editor. The suspicion arises that the latter's role may have been greater than in the case of the previous editions, especially since Burdon himself was a man of letters, the author of nowadays completely forgotten works on literature, politics, and philosophy. But it seems that even if this were the case, if Burdon suggested certain ideas to Boruwłaski (perhaps copying the account of exotic travels from somewhere?), both the general concept and the final shape of the memoirs were ultimately the latter's decisions. Still, we have to conclude that these were not very good decisions. Despite the richer content, the last version of the memoirs is a significantly less successful work than the first. Essentially the only interesting fragments recount his long stay in Ireland, described colourfully, vividly, and with sympathy, although John Powell is undoubtedly right in suspecting the author of having greatly embellished this story as well.[15] Elsewhere, the excessive textbook-style information about countries he truly or allegedly visited grows tedious, the anecdotes sometimes give the impression of having been thought up especially to impress readers (although perhaps this is being unfair to the author), and above all the book lacks what lent value to the earlier editions – the personal stamp of the author. And so we might conclude here: there were many travellers who described their adventures, but there was only one Boruwłaski.

---

[15] J.S. Powell, op. cit., p. 1.

Conclusion

The lengthy trip Boruwłaski's story takes us on, across the Europe of the turn of the eighteenth and nineteenth centuries, is undoubtedly a curious journey. That is because the little count himself was a very unusual traveller. To put it harshly, he roamed country after country not with the ordinary traveller's aim of seeing and experiencing things but to himself be seen and admired there, to find new audiences to exhibit himself before.

Biographies typically go to great lengths to depict their subject's life as it fits in with the broader milieu they belonged to, the society they were a member of, the country they were a citizen of. But Boruwłaski's case is an exception: he did not belong anywhere, and for a significant portion of his life he remained outside all social and national structures. As we have seen in the foregoing, he was a kind of Gulliver trapped in the land of giants (once again I borrow a metaphor from Boruwłaski himself), to some extent always an outsider everywhere, regardless of what social circle he found himself in. He fully realised this status himself, writing: 'my stature has irrevocably excluded me from the common circle of society.' Unlike Swift's character, he was even deprived of any chance to return home from his voyaging, to come back to his rightful place in the end. Rather, Boruwłaski was a Gulliver doomed to live in Brobdingnag his entire life.

Although Boruwłaski's writings do not quite share the fictional captain's acute perceptiveness and acumen, his recounting of his life story nevertheless does speak volumes about the world he knew first-hand, as viewed from the perspective 'of a being, stamped by nature herself on the coin of the marvellous' – especially the world of Enlightenment-age elite society and the Salons. The insight Boruwłaski offers us into certain little-known aspects of the culture of that society's upper echelons is not so much evident in his descriptions as it is simply demonstrated by his very existence.

It is a kind of paradox that a man who was denied a normal place among normal society was at the same time allowed to access the 'very best society' of the day, access he never could have enjoyed had he been of normal height.

However, that access came on specific terms and conditions. He did his utmost to live up to those expectations and he never criticised his 'benefactors.' But despite that, Boruwłaski's perspective on the elite of his day yields us a picture that its representatives would presumably not have been entirely proud of or found very flattering. This is a picture of people well-educated in the culture of their epoch, many of them even refined aestheticians and subtle intellectuals, who were nevertheless ceaselessly following fashion and seeking sensation, intrigued by deformities and oddities and fascinated by otherness, while at the same time being somewhat ashamed of that fascination as being at odds with the very aesthetic ideals they professed. It is a picture of people who turn out to be on the one hand 'sensitive' and romantic, often waxing sentimental at poor little Joujou's lot in life, while on the other remaining brutally indifferent to his real feelings and needs. And, above all, of people who were filled with a sense of own their boundless superiority over this talking toy, this animated miracle of nature, who were convinced that they could and even should treat him like an object or at best like a pleasant pet animal, and who became sincerely outraged when he dared to oppose them.

The memoirs also leave us with a memorable image of Joujou/Gulliver himself, a sensitive and intelligent man painfully aware of his own predicament, struggling his whole life to liberate himself from the roles forced upon him by society and by nature, even at the price of losing his safe harbour in Humiecka's salon. A playing of the salons, leading an adventurer's lifestyle despite his own wishes, a man who was never 'at home' and yet, we must admit, who was always able to adapt. A man shaped and educated by the very society that rejected him, which taught him not only the sophisticated suave demanded by the salons but also flexibility, the ability to keep his wits about him in any situation. A Gulliver whose story at long, long last did draw to a happy end – he may not have sailed back to his home port (indeed he had none), but through his own tenacity, intelligence, personal charm, and also thanks to human kindness he did ultimately find a place for himself. This was a place different in every respect from both the one in which he was born and the one which had educated him: it was among the cultural and intellectual elite and the nobility of a small English town and its vicinity that he found a place to call home, a place that accepted him. What then remained of his former high-society identity was a lingering legend that had already formed in the eighteenth century and would prove to be highly resilient – distant echoes can even be found on the Internet today.

Boruwłaski's life story and his memoirs may not, admittedly, be seen as the stuff of history with a capital 'H,' but the present biographical essay has striven to show that they do nevertheless merit closer investigation – on account of both Boruwłaski's captivating personality and the fresh and interesting perspective he gives us on the European society of his era.

Bibliography

Manuscript Sources

Archiwum Główne Akt Dawnych
[Polish Central Archives of Historical Records], Warsaw

Archiwum Królestwa Polskiego 82 (Correspondence of Franciszek Bukaty with
  Departament Interesów Cudzoziemskich of Rada Nieustająca).
Zbiory Muzeum Narodowego 79 (Correspondence of Franciszek Bukaty).

Biblioteka Czartoryskich [Czartoryski Library] Kraków

MS 924, Polish correspondence of Stanisław Augustus.
MS 2798, three letters of Joseph Boruwlaski to Emma George, 1826.

British Library

MS Add. 47563, correspondence of Charles James Fox.

Durham University Library

MS Add. 180, letter of Joseph Boruwlaski to Miss Mary Ebdon, 20 May 1818.
S.R. Cabinet C1, letter of Joseph Boruwlaski to the editors of his Memoirs,
  27 May 1818.

Favre Family collection

Letters of Georgiana Fanny Boruwłaska-Kean to her daughter Julie Alfonsine
  Malenfant-Favre (1842–1852).

Printed Primary Sources

Boruwlaski's Memoirs

Mémoires du célèbre nain Joseph Boruwlaski gentilhomme polonois, écrits par lui même en français et traduit en anglais par Des Carrières, London, 1788.

Leben des bekannten Zwerges Joseph Boruwlaski, eines polnischen Edelmans. Aus dem Englischen [übersetzt C.A. Wichmann], Leipzig, 1790.

Mémoires du célèbre nain Joseph Boruwlaski gentilhomme polonois, écrits par lui même, revus, corrigés et augmentés. Birmingham: J. Thompson, 1792.

A Second Edition of the Memoirs of the Celebrated Dwarf Joseph Boruwlaski, a Polish Gentleman, carefully revised and corrected, and translated from the French by Mr S. Freeman. Birmingham: J. Thompson, 1792.

Memoirs of the Celebrated Dwarf Joseph Boruwlaski, a Polish Gentleman, translated from the original French, and carefully revised and corrected. Kelso: James Ballantyne, 1801.

Memoirs of Count Boruwlaski: containing a sketch of his travels, with an account at the different courts of Europe written by himself, corrected by Mr Burdon. Durham: F. Humble, 1820.

The Life and Love Letters of a Dwarf, ed. H.R. Heatley. London, Ibister & Co, 1902.

Other Printed Primary Sources

Catalogue of Furniture, Books and other Effects of the Late Celebreted Polish Dwarf Count Boruwlaski, to be sold by auction, the 29th Day of November, 1838.

Correspondence inédite du roi Stanislas Auguste Poniatowski et de Mme Geoffrin (1764–1777), ed. Ch. de Mouy, Paris, 1875.

Encyclopédie, ou dictionnaire raisonné des sciences, des arts et des métiers, vol. 11, Neuchâtel, 1765.

Granger, W. (ed.). *The New Wonderful Museum.* London, Hogg & Co, 1804.

Hunt, M. 'Account of her early life by Margaret Hunt' in *A Raine Miscellany,* ed. by Angela Marsden, The publications of the Surtees Society, vol. 200, 1991.

Hutton, C. 'A Memoir of the Celebrated Dwarf Joseph Boruwlaski', *Bentley's Miscellany*, vol. 17, 1845.

Koblański, J. 'Oda na maski krakowskie w karnawał 1773 w bandzie J.W. Humieckiej, Miecznikowej Koronnej', in *Wiersze Józefa Koblańskiego i Stanisława Szczęsnego Potockiego zapomnianych poetów Oświecenia*, ed. E. Aleksandrowska. Ossolineum, Wrocław, 1980.

Lach-Szyrma, K. *Anglia i Szkocja. Przypomnienia z podróży roku 1820–1824 odbytej*. ed. P. Hertz. Warsaw, PIW, 1981.

Lyson, D. *Lyson's Colletanea, or a collection of advertisement and paragraphs from the newspapers relating to various subjects, vol. 1: Public exhibitions and places of amusement.*

Mathews, A. *Memoirs of Charles Mathews Comedian*, vol. 3, London, 1839.

Niemcewicz, J.U. *Pamiętniki czasów moich*, ed. J. Dihm, Warszawa, PIW, 1957

Ross, M. *A historical and Descriptive View of the City of Durham: Comprising an Account of its Cathedral, Churches, chapels, Castle, Bridges, County Court and other public Buildings; its Institutions, civil government etc. etc..* Newcastle-upon-Tyne, John Sykes, 1834.

'Royal Arcade Exhibition of Paintings, Drawings, and Sculpture' [Newcastle, n. d. leaflet].

Sibbald, S. *The Memoirs of Susan Sibbald (1783–1812)*, ed. by her great-grandson Francis Paget Hett, s. l., J. Lane, 1926.

A Series of Original Portraits and Caricature Etchings, by late John Kay [.] with Biographical Sketches and Illustrative Anecdotes, vol. 1, Edinburgh, 1837.

Tressan, L.E. de. *Mémoire envoyé à l'Académie Royale des Sciences par M. le Comte*. Paris, 1760.

The Volunteer; New Sonata for the Pianoforte or Harpsichord, composed by Count Joseph Boruwlaski, dedicated to the Hon. Mrs Buchanan, Edinburgh. S. l. [1804?]

Newspapers and Periodicals

Annual Register, 13.05.1761.
Bath Chronicle, 07.08.1788; 24.01.1805.
Craftsman, 03.08.1821.

Durham Chronicle, 08.09.1837.
Durham County Advertiser, 20.05.1820; 08.09.1837.
Gazetteer, 19.10.1786; 31.12.1759.
Gloucester Journal, 04.06.1804.
London Magazine, April 1760.
Morning Herald, 06.05.1786; 06.05.1783.
Morning Post, 30.05.1782.
Newcastle Chronicle, 27.06.1801; 29.08.1801.
Newcastle Courant, 28.12.1799.
Oxford Journal, 06.12.1788.
The Times, 13.09.1837.
Watchman, 27.09.1837.

Secondary Sources

Benedict, B. 'Displaying Difference: Curious Count Boruwlaski and the Staging of Class Identity', *Eighteenth-Century Life*, vol. 30, no. 3, summer 2006, p. 78–106.

Biographia Curiosa or Memoirs of Remarkable Characters of the Reign of George the Third, collected by George Smeeton and others, London, J. Robins & Co., 1822.

Biographie universelle et portative des contemporains, ed. C.A. Vieilh de Boisjoslin, Paris, 1830.

Carlton, C.M. *The Monumental Inscriptions of the Cathedral, Parish Churches and cemeteries of the City of Durham*, Durham, W. Ainsley & Bro., 1880.

Dictionary of National Biographies, ed. L. Stephen, London, Smith, Elder & Co.,1885.

Encyklopedia powszechna Orgelbranda, Warsaw, vol. 2, 1898.

Evans, H. and M. *John Kay of Edinburgh: Barber, miniaturist and Social Commentator*, Aberdeen, Impulse Publications, 1973.

Fabiani, B. *Niziołki, łokietki, karlikowie*, Warsaw, PIW, 1980.

Foreman, A. *Georgiana, Duchess of Devonshire*, 1st edn, London, Harper Collins, 1998.

Gaber, S. *L'entourage polonais du roi Stanislas Leszczyński à Lunéville*, Nancy, 1972.

Gould, R.F. 'Freemasonry in Cheshire', *Ars Quatuor Coronatorum*, 15, 1902.

Heron, T. *The Little Count Joseph Boruwlaski*, City of Durham, 1986.

K.T.H. [Klementyna z *Tańskich* Hoffmanowa], Józef Borusławski, *Przyjaciel Ludu*, vol. 5, Leszno, 1838.

Notes and Queries, May, 1856; August, 1857.

Rozmaitości, Lwów, no. 24, 1845.

Leroi, A.M. *Mutants: on the form, varieties and errors of the human Body*, London: HarperCollins, 2003.

Johnson, M. 'Boruwlaski, Joseph, styled Count Boruwlaski (1739–1837)', *Oxford Dictionary of National Biography*, online edn, Oxford University Press, Sept 2004.

Polski Słownik Biograficzny, vol. 2, Kraków, PAU, 1937.

Powell, J.S. *Joseph Boruwlaski his Visit to Portarlington 1795*, York, no date.

Ryba, J. *Uwodzicielskie oblicza Oświecenia*, Katowice, Wydawnictwo Naukowe Śląsk, 1994.

Słowiński, M. *Błazen. Dzieje motywu i postaci*, Warszawa, "Prolog", 1993.

Strand Magazine, vol. 8, July–December 1894.

Wilson, Henry. *Wonderful Characters*, vol. 3, London, 1822.

Wood, F.J. *Giants and Dwarfs*, London, Bentley, 1868.

Wasylewski, S. *Romans prababki*, Lwów, Wydawnictwo Polskie, 1920.

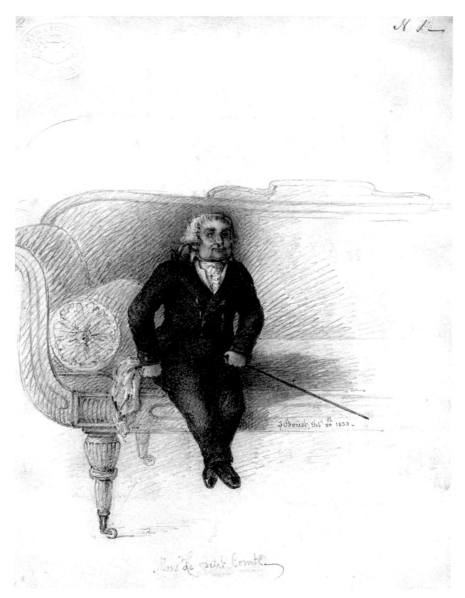

Plate 1   Joseph Boruwłaski on the sofa, sketch, Joseph Bouet, Feb. 20th
1833, Durham University Library, Misc. 1985: Bouet Album. MSS
1300/1.

MEMOIRS

OF THE

CELEBRATED DWARF,

JOSEPH BORUWLASKI,

A POLISH GENTLEMAN;

CONTAINING

A faithful and curious Account of his BIRTH, EDU-
CATION, MARRIAGE, TRAVELS and VOYAGES;

WRITTEN BY HIMSELF;

Translated from the French

By Mr. DES CARRIERES.

With a Copper-plate Engraving, wherein he is represented in a
Family-Scene.

LONDON, 1788.

Plate 2   Boruwłaski's Memoirs, 1st edition, frontispiece by William Hincks and title page

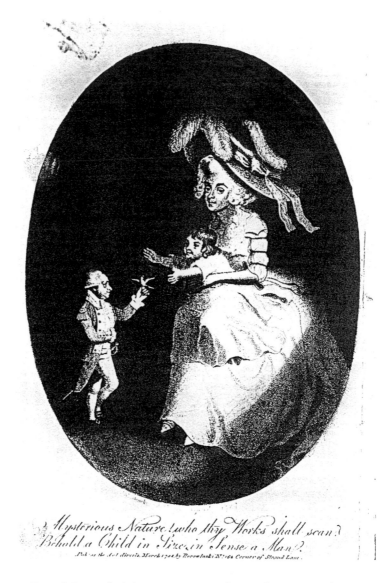

Mysterious Nature! who thy Works shall scan?
Behold a Child in Size, in Sense a Man?

Pub. as the Act directs, March 1788 by Boruwlaski, N.º 164 Corner of Strand Lane.

Plate 2a   Detail, Boruwłaski's Memoirs, 1st edition, frontispiece by William Hincks

MEMOIRS

OF

COUNT BORUWLASKI:

CONTAINING

A SKETCH OF HIS TRAVELS,

WITH

AN ACCOUNT OF HIS RECEPTION

AT THE DIFFERENT

COURTS OF EUROPE,

&c. &c.

WRITTEN BY HIMSELF.

DURHAM:

PRINTED BY FRANCIS HUMBLE AND CO,
AND SOLD BY BALDWIN, CRADOCK, AND JOY, LONDON; ANDREWS,
DURHAM; AND BY THE BOOKSELLERS IN NEWCASTLE,
SUNDERLAND, NORTH AND SOUTH SHIELDS,
STOCKTON, DARLINGTON, ETC.

1820.

Plate 3   Boruwłaski's Memoirs, ed. 1820, frontispiece by Joseph Bouet and title page

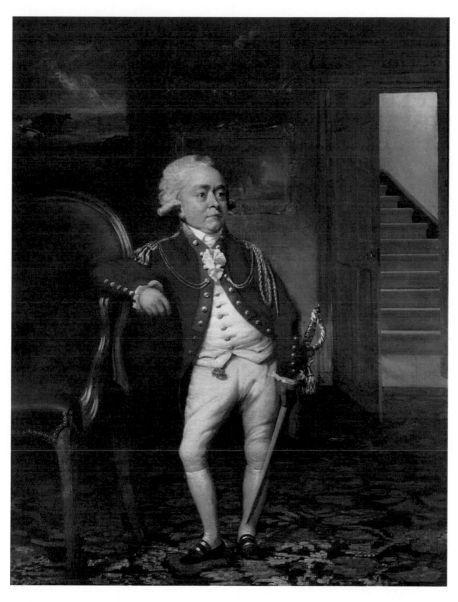

Plate 4   Joseph Boruwłaski, portrait, Philip Reinagle, The Royal College of
         Surgeons

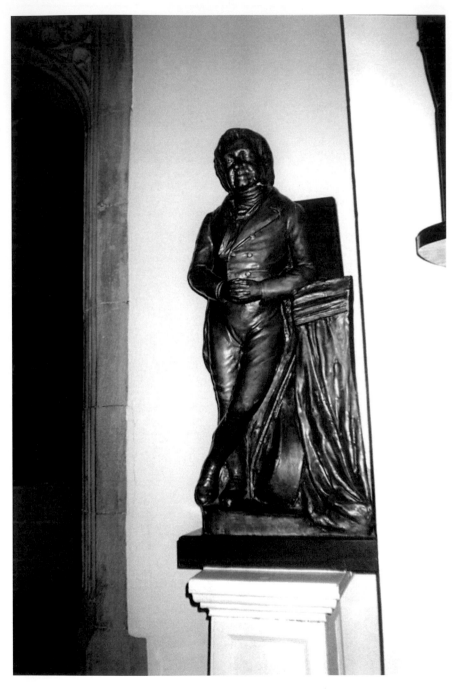

Plate 5   Joseph Boruwłaski, statue, Joseph Bonomi, Town Hall Durham

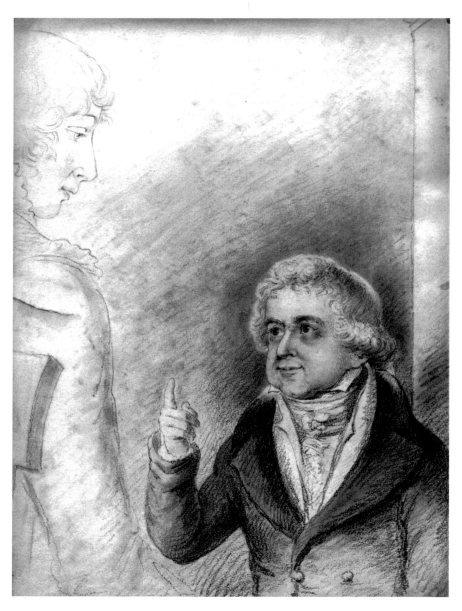

Plate 6   Joseph Boruwłaski, sketch, Joseph Bouet, Durham University Library, Misc. 1985: Bouet Album

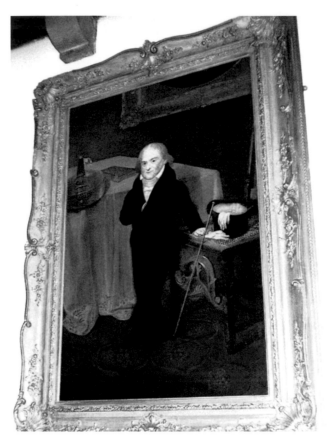

Plate 7   Joseph Boruwłaski, portrait, Edmund Hastings, Town Hall Durham

A SECOND EDITION OF

THE MEMOIRS

OF THE

Celebrated Dwarf,

JOSEPH BORUWLASKI,

A POLISH GENTLEMAN.

Containing

A faithful and curious Account

OF

HIS BIRTH, EDUCATION, MARRIAGE, TRAVELS,
AND VOYAGES.

WRITTEN BY HIMSELF; AND CAREFULLY
REVISED AND CORRECTED.

And tranſlated from the French by Mr. S. Freeman.

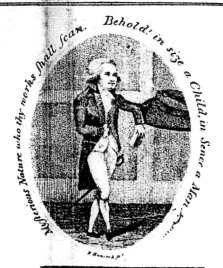

Birmingham.

PRINTED BY J. THOMPSON.

1792.

Plate 8   Boruwłaski's Memoirs, 2nd ed., title page

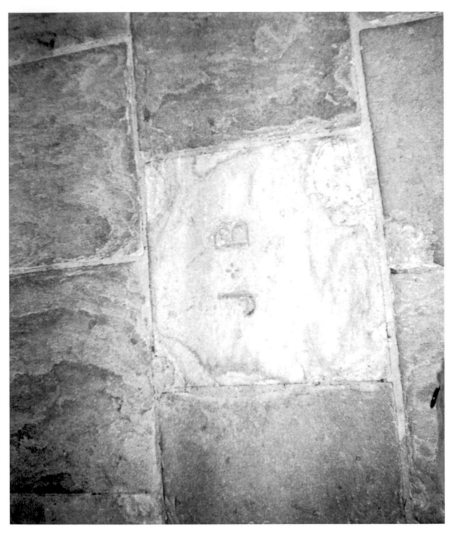

Plate 9   Tombstone of Boruwłaski, Durham Cathedral

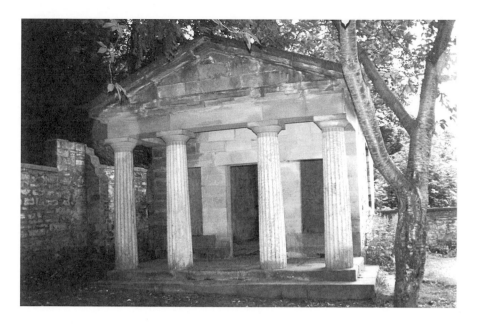

Plate 10   'Boruwłaski's house', Durham

COUNT BORUWLASKI

Has the Honor of informing the Public, that his MEMOIRS, written by himself, and dedicated, by Permission, to His ROYAL HIGHNESS THE PRINCE REGENT, are ready for the Press, and will be published as soon as a sufficient Number of Subscribers shall be obtained to defray the Expence of Printing.   Price to Subscribers, 12s.—to Non-Subscribers, 15s.

Subscribers' Names received by Mr. CHARNLEY, Bookseller, Newcastle, and Mr. ANDREWS, Bookseller, Durham.

Printed by F. Humble & Co. Durham.

Plate 11   Boruwłaski's Memoirs announcement, 1820

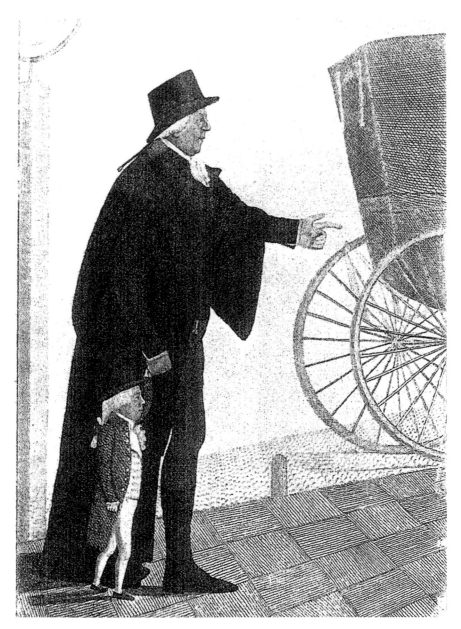

Plate 12   Boruwłaski with Neil Fergusson, copperplate, John Kay, in: Hilary
and Mary Evans, *John Kay of Edinburg. Barber, miniaturist and
Social Commentator*, Aberdeen, Impulse Publications, 1973, il. 71

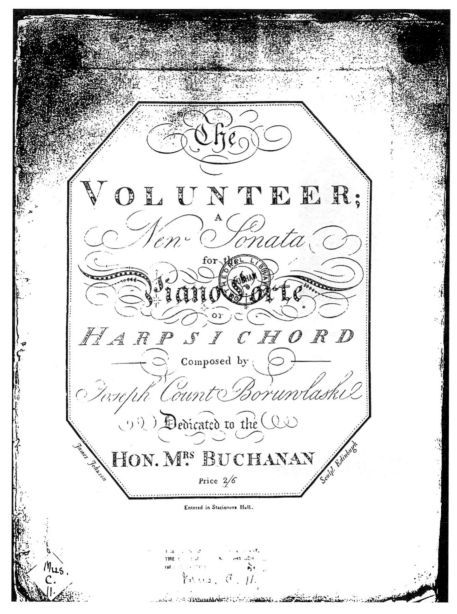

Plate 13   Joseph Boruwłaski's composition 'The Volunteer', Edinburgh, no
date, Durham Cathedral Library, Mus. C. 11

Gentlemen

I had the pleasure to receive your kind letter, which informed me that the Rev.d M.r Kitchinman had appointed M.r Wolstenholme to take the names of Subscribers. I must however beg the favour that you will also honour me with receiving names. for which purpose you were so kind as to offer your trouble. It will be ne.cessary to publish the advertisement of which I send you a copy with this Letter. I remain

Durham May 27   Gentlemen

1818.   your most Obliged obedient

Servant

Joseph Boruwłaski

Plate 14   Boruwłaski's letter to the editor, Durham University Library, SR Cab C1 1818

MS942.8178218
Add. MS 180

May 20
1818

Dear Madam

I have the pleasure to informed you of my saf arrival to London, but unhappely I found my Dear M.r Burdon not quait to my satisfaction wee and I think he most remaind much longer in London, and probably will not come at all to the northe, so I will returne mayself to Durham. before that time I bag of you to present my best Complements to My good frend Miss Eliza Ebdon also Rev.d M.r Ebdon and M.r Ebdon; now I most Conclude for this time with truth and sincere affection to be

Madam your most humble most

Obedient Servand

Joseph Boruwłaski

Plate 15   Boruwłaski's letter to Mary Ebdon, Durham University Library, Add. Ms 180

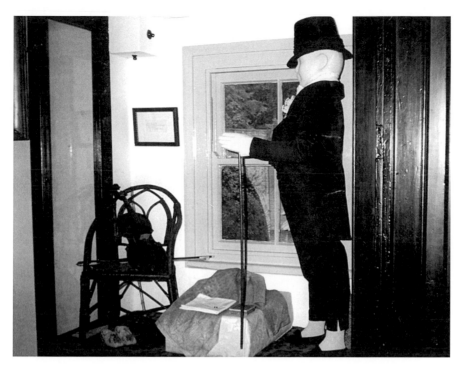

Plate 16   Boruwłaski's clothes and belongings, Town Hall Durham

THAT ASTONISHING PHENOMENON,

Sieur BORUWLASKI,

The celebrated MAN in MINIATURE,

(Whose Age is 48 Years, and his Height Three Feet Three Inches,)

Respectfully acquaints the GENTRY and PUBLIC in general,

That he will receive Company

At his Apartments, No. 163, near the NEW CHURCH,
STRAND.

Every Day, from TEN in the Morning till THREE in the Afternoon,
And from FIVE in the Afternoon till NINE in the Evening.

Admittance, One Shilling each Person.

Plate 17   Boruwłaski's announcement, London 1787, British Library, *Daniel Lyson's Collectanea or a collection of advertisement and paragraphs from the newspaper relating to various subjects, vol. 1: Public exhibitions and places of amusement*

BRISTOL, *March* 1, 1790.

Sieur Boruwlaſki,

THE CELEBRATED

POLISH LILLIPUTIAN,

NOT unmindful of the FAVORS he has heretofore received from the LADIES and GENTLEMEN of BRISTOL, and its ENVIRONS, feels it incumbent on him to pay his Reſpects to them once more, before his Departure for the CONTINENT, which he purpoſes taking in a very ſhort Time.——He therefore reſpectfully informs thoſe who may be diſpoſed to honour him with their Company during his ſhort Stay in BRIS-TOL,—That he has taken an APARTMENT

At Mr. VANDYKE's, No. 6, Corner of *Denmark-ſtreet*, St. *Auguſtine's-Back,*

(☞ The Door in *Denmark-Street,*)

WHERE

FOR A FEW DAYS ONLY,

He ſhall be happy to receive their Viſits from Ten in the Morning till Three, and from Four till Eight.

⁂ Admiſſion ONE SHILLING.

Children admitted at HALF PRICE.

Plate 18   Boruwłaski's announcement, Bristol 1790, British Library *Daniel Lyson's Collectanea or a collection of advertisement and paragraphs from the newspaper relating to various subjects, vol. 1: Public exhibitions and places of amusement*

ROYAL ARCADE EXHIBITION

OF

PAINTINGS, DRAWINGS, AND SCULPTURE.

FIRST ROOM.—PAINTINGS.

No. 10. A BATTLE SCENE, BY BORGOGNONE.

" This picture is powerfully painted, with rapid and vigorous handling.

" This Artist was born in 1621. His battle-pieces are painted with uncommon spirit, and display the ardour of a mind, delighted with the scene upon which it was engaged. 'In beholding his pictures,' says an intelligent writer, 'we seem to hear the shouts of war, the neighing of the horses, and cries of the wounded.' He died in Rome, in 1676."

SECOND ROOM.—SCULPTURE.

No. 27, STATUE OF COUNT BORUWLASKI,

(SIZE OF LIFE—3 FEET 2 INCHES.)

In the 90th year of his age, and in the form of dress which he wore, on being presented to his late Majesty, George the Fourth, modelled at the Count's residence, Durham, March 8th, 1832, by D. Dunbar.

" Count Boruwlaski was the son of a Polish Nobleman attached to the fortunes of King Stanislaus, who lost his property in consequence of that attachment, and who had six children, three dwarfs, and three well grown. What is singular enough, they were born alternately, a big one and a little one, though both parents were of the common size. The little Count's youngest sister was much less than him, but died at the age of 23. The Count continued to grow till he was about 30, when his height was 3 feet 2 inches. He never experienced any sickness, but lived in a polite and affluent manner, under the patronage of a lady, a friend of the family, till love, at the age of 41, intruded into his little peaceful bosom, and involved him in matrimony, care, and perplexity. The lady he chose was of his own country, but of French extraction, and the middle size. They have three children, all girls, and none of them likely to be dwarfs. To provide for a family now became an object big with difficulty, requiring all the exertion of his powers (which could promise but little) and his talents, of which music alone afforded any view of profit. He plays extremely well upon the guitar ; and by having concerts in several of the principal cities in Germany, he raised temporary supplies.

" At Vienna he was persuaded to turn his thoughts to England, where it was believed the public curiosity might in a little time benefit him sufficiently to enable him to live independently in so cheap a country as Poland. He was furnished by very respectable friends with recommendations to several of the most distinguished characters in this kingdom, the Duchess of Devonshire, Rutland, &c., whose kind patronage he is not backward to acknowledge. He was advised to let himself be seen as a curiosity, and the price of admission was fixed at a guinea. The number of his visitors of course was not very great. After a pretty long stay in London he went to Bath and Bristol ; visited Dublin, and some other parts of Ireland ; whence he returned by way of Liverpool, Manchester, and Birmingham, to London. He also visited Edinburgh, and some other towns in Scotland. In every place the Count acquired a number of friends. In reality, the ease and politeness of his manners and address please no less than the diminutive, yet elegant, proportions of his figure, astonish those who visit him. His person is pleasing and graceful, and his look manly and noble. He speaks French fluently, and English tolerably. He is remarkably lively and cheerful, though fitted for the most serious and rational conversation. Such is this wonderful little man—an object of curiosity really worthy the attention of the philosopher, the man of taste, and the anatomist. His life was published at Durham, written by himself, in 1820."—*Vide Encyclopædia Britannica.*

Open from Nine o'Clock till Dusk. Admission One Shilling.

W. Braz, Printer, Dean Street, Newcastle.

Plate 19   Announcement of sculpture exhibition with Boruwłaski's statue by David Dunbar

BORUWLASKI's BALL.

A numerous, select, and brilliant company graced Sieur Boruwlaski's Ball, at the Crown and Anchor on Friday last, and most complete was their gratifications.—With spirits inexhaustible, this wonderful little creature strained every nerve to give them pleasure. *Hic et ubique*, here, there, and every where, not an individual but enjoyed some moments of his conversation. With an ease and neatness of execution which would not have disgraced Vestris, he joined his Lady in the KOSAK, a dance replete with grace and variety. This elegant performance was received with an unanimous burst of applause, a very considerable share of which went most deservedly to Madame Boruwlaski. Their admiration was next heightened by some delicious airs on the guittar, which the little gentleman gave with exquisite neatness and taste. But the company were not yet satisfied; he could not so soon be parted with; a repetition of the Kosak was called for by the whole room—and the request granted with the utmost good humour. Thus with the introduction of minuets and the exhilarating country dance, the evening wore delightfully away, nor was the room cleared till one o'clock, when the company departed in raptures with their entertainment, and warm with zeal for the interests and welfare of the astonishing Being who had so essentially contributed to it. We applaud his intentions of making his next remove East of Temple Bar (before he finally quits the kingdom) and casting himself on the protection of the Citizens, whose taste and liberality we estimate at so high a rate, that we shall be much mistaken in our predictions, if he prove not a magnet of very considerably attractive powers.

Plate 20   Boruwłaski's advertisement, Morning Herald, June 2, 1788, British Library, *Daniel Lyson's Collectanea or a collection of advertisement and paragraphs from the newspaper relating to various subjects, vol.1: Public exhibitions and places of amusement*

CATALOGUE

OF

FURNITURE, BOOKS,

AND OTHER EFFECTS

OF THE

LATE CELEBRATED POLISH DWARF

COUNT BORUWLASKI,

TO BE SOLD BY AUCTION,

(BY MR. WALKER,)

AT THE ROOMS IN THE QUEEN'S COURT, NEAR THE
PUBLIC SALE AND EXHIBITION ROOM,
NORTH BAILEY, DURHAM,

On *THURSDAY, the 29th Day of NOVEMBER,* 1838.

The Sale to commence at Eleven o'clock.

DURHAM:

PRINTED BY G. WALKER, JUN., SADLER-STREET.

Price Two-Pence.

Plate 21   'Catalogue of Furniture, Books, and other effects of the late celebrated Polish dwarf Count Boruwłaski, to be sold by auction, (by Mr. Walker,) at the rooms in the Queen's Court, near the public sale and exhibition room, North Bailey, Durham, on Thursday, the 29th day of November, 1838', Durham University Library, XL 920B7 BOR

The Memoirs of the Celebrated Dwarf, Joseph Boruławski

Editorial note

The basis for this annotated edition is the first English publication of Boruwłaski's memoirs from 1788, translated by Jean Thomas Hérissant Des Carrières. This is the best English version in literary terms, the most personal one, and moreover it is the only edition that contains the whole of the correspondence between Joujou and Isalina.

Boruwłaski's/Des Carières original orthography and punctuation have been left intact, because they do not overly hamper the modern-day reader and in fact preserve a certain quaint flavour of the period. Modern-day readers are aided by quite extensive footnotes, mainly containing supplementary information about individuals and events referred to in the memoirs.

Added as a supplementary text at the end, meant to serve as a kind of illustration of the kind of attitudes that prevailed with respect to Boruwłaski, is a translation of the scholarly report on him delivered by the Count de Tressan to the French Royal Academy of Sciences (*Mémoire envoyé à l'Académie Royale des Sciences par M. le Comte de Tressan*, Paris 1760).

Memoirs of the Celebrated Dwarf Joseph Boruwłaski, a Polish Gentleman, containing a faithful and curious Account of his Birth, Education, Marriage, Travels and Voyages; written by himself; translated from the French by Mr Des Carrières, London 1788

To her Grace the Duchess of Devonshire.[1]

Madam,

no words can express the obligations I am under, not only for your unremitted favours conferred upon me from the very moment of my arrival in England, but also for the completion of them by your condescension, in permitting me to dedicate to your Grace these Memoirs, and thereby attempt, however feebly, to manifest my gratitude. On their reception in the world, entirely depend my future welfare and my family's support. Can I entertain the least doubt of their meeting with the general acceptance, when they are presented under your Grace's auspices and patronage? How flattering is the idea, how delightful is the prospect, to be indebt for all to Protectress, who, still more by her talents and internal qualities, than by the charms of external elegance, victoriously sways every heart.. But here I stop.. Though my feelings may be ever so lively, yet they cannot impart the talents which are wanting in me, and considering my inherent insufficiency, I must only admire in silence. I am with the most profound respect, Madam, Your Grace's most obedient, most dutiful and humble servant, Jos. Boruwlaski.

---

[1] Georgiana, Duchess of Devonshire (1757–1806, the daughter of Count John Spencer), married William Cavendish, Duke of Devonshire, in 1774.

Memoirs, &c.

It is so uncommon to find reason and sentiment, with noble and delicate affections, in a man whom nature, as it were, could not make up, and who in size has the appearance of a child, that, persuaded nobody would even take the trouble to cast an eye upon these Memoirs, I began to commit to paper some of the principal events of my life, by way of memorandums, for my own use, only to remind me of the different situations I had been in, to recall to my memory scenes too interesting, emotions too strong to die in oblivion. As the reflections which I shall have occasion to make can be interesting only to those who delight in following nature through all her different ways, who are wont to look upon beings of my stature as upon abortive half-grown individuals, kept far beneath other men, both in body and mind; and who, consequently, may be curious to see one of them assimilate himself to creatures of common size, as to his views, affections, passions and ideas; I should not have taken the liberty of presenting them to the public, had not persons, to whom I ought not to refuse any thing, imposed it upon me as a duty. May I be so happy, when I offer this tribute of my gratitude, as to convince them how deeply I felt the interest they took in my concerns.

I was born in the environs of Chaliez, capital of Pokucia in Polish Russia[2] in November 1739. My parents were of the middle size; they had six children, five sons, and one daughter; and by one of those freaks of nature, which it is impossible to account for, or perhaps to find another instance of in the annals of the human species, three of these children grew to above the middle stature, whilst the two others, like myself, reached only that of children in general at the age of four or five years.

I am the third of this astonishing family. My eldest brother, who at this time is about sixty, is near three inches taller than I am. He has constantly enjoyed a robust constitution, and has still strength and vigour much above his size and age. He has lived a long time with the Castelane Inowloska,[3] who honours him with her esteem and bounty; and finding in him ability and sense enough, has intrusted him with the stewardship and management of her affairs.

---

[2] Halicz, a town on the Dniester River in the Pokucie region in the south-east of the Polish-Lithuanian Republic, the so-called 'Polish Russia' or Ruthenia (now Halych in Ukraine).

[3] Most likely the wife of Bogusław Ustrzycki, Castellan of Inowlódz in 1756–1785.

My second brother was of a weak and delicate frame; he died at twenty-six, being at the time five feet ten inches high. Those who came into the world after me, were alternately tall and short: among them was a female, who died of the small-pox at the age of twenty-two. She was at that time only two feet two inches high, and to lovely figure united an admirably well proportioned shape.

It was easy to judge from the very instant of my birth, that I should be extremely short, being at the time only eight inches; yet, notwithstanding this diminutive proportion, I was neither weak nor puny: on contrary, my mother, who suckled me, has often declared that none of her children gave her less trouble. I walked, and was able to speak at about the age common to other infants, and my growth was progressively as follows:

At one year I was	11 inches high, English measure.
At three	–1 foot 2 inches
At six	–1 - 5
At ten	–1 - 9
At fifteen	–2 feet 1
At twenty	–2 - 4
At twenty-five	–2 - 11
At thirty	–3 - 3

This is the size at which I remained fixed, without having afterwards increased half a quarter of an inch; by which the assertion of some naturalists proves false, viz. that Dwarfs grow during all their life-time. If this instance were insufficient, I could cite that of my brother, who, like me, grew 'till thirty; and like me, at that age, ceased to grow taller.

I had scarcely entered my ninth year when my father died, and left my mother with six children, and very small share in the favours of fortune: a circumstance to which I am indebted for the part I have since acted in the world. Had it not been so, I undoubtedly should have lived obscure and unknown, buried in a province on the banks of Nieper;[4] and perhaps I had been happier.

---

[4] Meaning the Dnieper River – but apparently an error: the author himself indicates that he comes from the region of Pokucia, which lies on the Dniester River, not on the even more easterly Dnieper. Possibly an intentional error, with the author opting to mention the much larger and better-known Dnieper instead.

A friend of my mother, the Starostina de Caorliz,[5] shewed me much affection, and often had solicited my parents to commit my education to her care. She availed herself of the embarrassed circumstances of our family, to repeat her kind offers to my mother, who thought it might prove grievous to her, yielded to the desire of making me happy; and insisting no longer on keeping me at home, consented, but not without tears, to part with me; and Lady de Caorliz took me to her estate, which was not very far from my mother's abode.

We had no sooner arrived there, than the Starostina, eager to fulfill her promises to my mother, bestowed upon me all the care that my age required. I lived with her four years; and the fondness of my benefactress no way diminishing, I was likely to be fixed for ever with her, when an unexpected event changed the face of things.

Lady de Caorliz was a widow, somewhat advanced in years, but still fresh-coloured and graceful: besides, she enjoyed a large fortune. The Count of Tarnow,[6] whom some affairs had drawn to the neighborhood, paid his court to her, and I soon perceived she highly distinguished him above all the persons who composed her society. She became pensive and absent; she seemed no longer amused with my little prattling, and I was not surprised at seeing Hymen unite these two lovers. Not was I unconscious of all the alteration my situation would suffer by their marriage. I felt that my protectress, by taking a husband, had given herself a master, that, should I chance to displease him, I was in danger of being so much the more embarrassed, as my family affairs, which were totally overthrown, left no resource. Therefore I considered it as my duty to double my efforts, that I might render myself agreeable to the husband of my benefactress; and I think I should have succeeded, had not a new event disappointed me, and given rise to other projects.

Some months after their marriage, the Countess de Tarnow thought she was pregnant. The joy of this happy couple may be easily conceived. They were

---

[5]   Helena Stadnicka, née Morska, by her second husband Tarnowska (–1771); the title used by Boruwłaski refers not to a surname but to the office held by her first husband Stadnicki, who was starosta of the town of Kahorlik (now Kaharlyk) in the Kiev district.

[6]   Jan Jacek Tarnowski (1729–1808) – genealogies list 1758 as the date of Stadnicka's marriage to Tarnowski, whereas Boruwłaski's account indicates that it took place somewhat earlier. It is hard to ascertain the truth here, but it should be borne in mind that Boruwłaski's dating is frequently off the mark.

congratulated on this occasion by all their friends, among whom they reckoned Countess Humieska.[7] This lady, who is descended from one of the most ancient families in Poland, is held in the highest rank in that country, not more for her birth and wealth, than for her personal qualities. Her estate being situated near the seat of Starostina, she had frequented opportunities of seeing me, and seemed to have some affection for me, as she often expressed what pleasure she should have, if I came to live with her at Warsaw. My answers to her obliging offers gained me her friendship more and more; nay, from that moment, she had very likely formed the project to ask me of the Countess de Tarnow, and only waited for a favourable opportunity.

The pretended pregnancy of my protectress, supplied the Countess Humieska with pretext. Being one day with the new married couple, she artfully took an opportunity of introducing the dangers pregnant women are exposed to, and after having instanced many accidents which some ladies of her acquaintance had experienced, stooped towards the Count, and asked him, loud enough to be heard, whether he did not fear some danger for his lady from my continually being under her eyes, and if that would not affect the child she was big with.

At such a question the couple started, and looked silently at each other. The Countess Humieska seeing them moved, set forth as an additional proof, an infinite number of facts calculated to increase their uneasiness; advised them to part with me; and offered, if they resolved to follow her advice, to take care of me, promising to do her best to make me happy.

Whether the new couple were really alarmed, or whether they feared to disoblige such a lady as the Countess, they but weakly resisted, and declared they left it to my decision. I was absent: the servant who came to fetch me, informed me of what had passed. I entered the apartment, quite prepared with my answer, and assured the Countess, that, if the Lady de Tarnow, whose bounty rendered her the mistress of my fate, deigned to grant me her consent, I should deem myself happy to live under the protection of the Countess, and would follow my inclination as much as my duty, by earnestly endeavouring to deserve her kindness.

---

[7]   Anna Humiecka, the widow of Józef Humiecki (died 1754), who held the rank of Sword-Bearer of the Polish Crown. Being née Rzewuska (the daughter of Michał Rzewuski), from one of the best families in Poland, she was also a descendant of the Sobieski royal family.

The Countess Humieska seemed overjoyed at my consent: 'I am very glad,' said she, 'my dear Joujou, (for so they called me), to see you have no reluctance to come and live with me.' Then addressing the Count and Countess de Tarnow: 'You cannot retract,' she said, 'I have your word and that of Joujou.' The remainder of the visit passed in compliments and our departure was fixed for a few days after.

Although I was under great obligations to the Countess de Tarnow, yet I own that I was soon easily reconciled to my separation from her. For this I hope I shall be forgiven, on considering that I was but fifteen, having my head filled with the lively picture my protectress had given me of the pleasures I should enjoy at her house. She carried me to her estate, at Rychty in Podolia,[8] where we stayed six months; and her Ladyship, whose design was to see Germany and France, desiring to have me with her. I felt the greatest pleasure in the flattering idea I entertained of those travels. After some indispensable preparations, we set out for Vienna.

The reader, perhaps, will not be displeased to know the manner of travelling in Poland. At that time I was too young, and my mind to little improved to be much impressed with it; but it has caused me since to make many sad reflections.

Let it be first imagined, that on the roads there are neither inns or public-houses of any kind to be found, nor any decent resort wherein the traveller can meet with the least conveniency; that consequently he is obliged to carry with him his kitchen-furniture, household-goods and provisions; that there he sees nothing in the country he goes through, but some sorry villages, chiefly inhabited by Jews; that in the dwelling of those poor wretches, a kind of barn where men and animals live promiscuously, Polish travellers take their abode; that they take care to send before them some servants, who choosing the place they think most convenient, drive the inhabitants out of it, often with heavy lashes, and even use the same violence sometimes upon other travellers, who, inferior in rank, dare not contend for the spot; that servants being in possession of the place, cover the walls with hangings, set up beds and the furniture they have brought; so that the masters, when they arrive, find their lodgings ready and decently furnished.

---

[8]   Rychty, a small town at south-east of Polish-Lithuanian Republic (now Richta in Ukraine). In the eighteenth century, Rychty Castle was in the possession of the Humiecki family.

It may be easily imagined, that such insolent servants spare not the poultry and vegetables of the poor Jews, who, whilst their property is thus disposed of, seek for refuge in some neighbouring hovels, wherein they impatiently wait for the departure of those troublesome guests, that they may return to their home again.

After some days of very fatiguing travel, and a dull stay for some months at Leopold,[9] we reached Vienna; where the report of our arrival was no sooner spread, than we were visited, invited and entertained with the utmost eagerness. Soon after we had the honour to be presented to her Imperial Majesty the Queen of Hungary,[10] who was graciously pleased to say, that I exceed by far all that she had heard of me, and that I was one of the most astonishing beings she had ever seen. At that time this great Princess was engaged in war with the King of Prussia,[11] and, by her firmness, courage and wisdom, had rendered herself no less terrible to her enemies than dear to her subjects. I had the honour to be one day in her apartment, when her courtiers complimented her on a victory obtained by her army, and every one extolled the advantageous consequences of it, so that, according to their account, the King of Prussia was like to be soon reduced to the last extremity.

The Empress, near whom I stood, asked me how the King of Prussia was looked upon in Poland, and what idea I entertained of that Prince. 'Madam,' I answered, 'I have not the honour to know him; but were I in his place, instead of losing my time in waging an useless war against you, I would come to Vienna, and pay may respects to you, deeming it a thousand times more glorious to gain your esteem and friendship, than to obtain the most complete victories over your troops.' Her Imperial Majesty seemed much pleased at my reply, hugged me in her arms, and said to my benefactress, she esteemed her very happy in having so pleasing a companion in her travels.

Another time, when, according to her desire, I had performed a Polish dance in the presence of this sovereign, she took me on her lap; and after having much caressed me, and asked many questions upon the manner how I spent my time,

---

9 Lwów, a major city in the south of the Polish-Lithuanian Republic (now Lviv in Ukraine).

10 Maria Theresa (1717–1780), ruler of Austria, Queen of Bohemia and Hungary (from 1740), and Empress as the wife of her husband, Emperor Francis Stephen (from 1745).

11 Frederick II Hohenzollern, known as Frederick the Great (1712–1786), King of Prussia (from 1740). This is a reference to the Seven Years War (1756–1763).

she wished to know what I found in Vienna most curious and interesting. I answered, I had seen there many things worthy of a traveller's admiration, but nothing seemed to me so extraordinary as what I beheld at that moment.

'And what is it?' said her Majesty

'It is,' replied I, 'to see so little a man on the lap of so great woman.'

This answer gained me new caresses. The Empress had on her finger a ring, upon which her cypher was set in brilliants, with the most exquisite workmanship. My hand being by chance locked in hers, I seemed to consider the ring attentively; which she perceived, and asked whether that cypher was pretty.

'I beg your Majesty's pardon,' replied I, 'it is not the ring I consider, but the hand, which I beseech you give me leave to kiss,' and with these words I took it to my lips.

The Empress seemed charmed at this little gallantry, and would have presented me with the ring which had caused it; but the circle proving too wide, she called to a young lady about five or six years old, who was then in the apartment, took from her finger a very fine diamond she wore, and put it on mine. This young person is now the Queen of France;[12] and it may be imagined I carefully preserve so precious a jewel.

It is easy to understand, that the kind notice of the Empress procured me the attention of her court; and I should be guilty of ingratitude, were I silent on the kindness his Excellency the Prince Kaunitz[13] shewed me. This great man, who at that time was ruling, as he still does, all affairs of the German empire, yet could find time to spend on small objects; and I may say, that the marks of friendship and interest he honoured me with, would have raised many jealousies, had not my size and mode of existence put me out of the common line. He called me his

---

[12]   Marie Antoinette (1755–1793), the daughter of Maria Theresa and the wife of Louis XVI (from 1770), Queen of France (from 1775), later sentenced to death during the French Revolution and beheaded at the guillotine. At the time of Boruwłaski's visit (late 1758/early 1759), born in November 1755 Marie Antoinette was younger than the author states, at only around three years old. Perhaps Maria Theresa gave Boruwłaski a ring from one of her somewhat older daughters (the one closest in age to Boruwłaski's account would have been Maria Carolina, born 1752), and the author simply ascribed it to the future Queen of France seeking to lend his tale more gravitas.

[13]   Wenzel Anton Kaunitz (1711–1794), Austrian statesman whom Maria Theresa appointed foreign minister in 1753 and chancellor soon thereafter, and who guided Austria's foreign policy for nearly 40 years.

little friend, pretending that my conversation both amused and interested him. In a word, on this journey, and on that I shall speak of hereafter, I had so much reason to be well pleased with his beneficence, that my only regret is, not to have any other means of testifying to him how deeply my heart is impressed with the remembrance of it.

Those, however, would be much mistaken, who should imagine that, seduced by the repeated kindnesses bestowed on me, or wholly devoted to the pleasures afforded me, I did not sometimes labour under painful feelings, or that I could always be unconscious of being, upon the whole, only looked upon by others as a doll, a little more perfect, it is true, and better organized than they commonly are, but, however, only as an animated toy. I remember, among other things, that one day in the apartment of my benefactress, when sitting in a corner at a little distance, and apparently paying no attention to the conversation, I heard they were speaking of me. One of the company having put the question, whether dwarfs posses the faculty of procreating? Another advanced, that if they have it, their children would grow to the common size; and the Countess Humieska acquainted her company with the state of my family, and in particular of my sister, whose size, she said, is still more extraordinary than that of Joujou. She added, she had often revolved in her own mind, how pleasant it would be to join these two little creatures, that the result might decide the question. I spare my readers the particulars of that conversation, which was carried very far, and only interrupted by my weeping bitterly; so strongly was I affected at the sort of contempt apparently implied in this project of uniting me with my sister; from which I thought I had to conclude, not only that they believed themselves entitled to dispose of me without my advice, but even looked upon me as a being merely physical, without morality, on whom they might try experiments of every kind. Somebody in the company perceiving my grief, wished to know the cause of it, which I persisted in concealing; and at length, not being able to stand against the solicitations of my benefactress, I declared it to her, who had much ado to console me, though she assured me she had never seriously thought on a marriage, of which the idea alone had shocked me so much. After all, I only relate this event to show, that though still very young during my first stay at Vienna, yet I was so far improved, and had acquired so much experience, as to feel all the impressions natural to those of my age.

We stayed at Vienna six months only, during which time my benefactress, availing herself of the opportunity, had me taught dancing by Mr. Angelini, the ballet-master to the Court, who since, by his eminent talents in his art, and his taste for literature, has rendered himself so famous.[14] Unluckily for me, being obliged to depart, I could not improve under his care as much as I wished: yet my benefactress could not forbear testifying, with raptures at what she called my progress, her gratitude to him, at our setting off for Bavaria.

Arrived at Munich, we were most graciously welcomed by his Electoral Highness,[15] and it seemed I excited no less curiosity there than at Vienna. During our stay, which was not long, and presents nothing peculiar, we spent our time in pleasures and entertainments. We left that place to repair to Lunéville, where Stanislaus Leckzinski [!], the titular king of Poland, held his court.[16]

I could not help being filled with respect, admiration and astonishment, at seeing this venerable old Prince, who, after such an agitated life, after having undergone the most fatal reverses of fortune, still preserved, at the age of eighty-years, all the faculties of his soul, and employed them with so much energy to promote the happiness of his new subjects. I was struck with his noble aspect, his mild and affable look, his serene and stately deportment. I immediately recollected the impression he made at first sight upon Charles XII.[17] It is known that this extraordinary monarch, after having conversed with him a quarter of an hour, said to the generals who composed his retenue: - This is the man who shall be king of Poland. It is known how Charles kept his word; how Stanislaus after the disgraces of his protector, saw himself stripped of that crown to which he had only aspired through his consciousness of the good he might do to his own

---

[14]   Casparo Angiolini (–1803), a dancer and choreographer (to use a modern term), Maria Theresa's court ballet master.

[15]   Maximilian III Joseph (1727–1777), Elector of Bavaria (from 1745).

[16]   Stanisław I Leszczyński (1677–1766), who had twice been King of Poland. The first time was during the Northern War, when he was essentially installed by the victorious troops of Charles XII of Sweden to succeed Augustus II as King of Poland in 1704; after the defeat of Swedes in 1709 he went into exile. He was elected king the second time in 1733; he lost the crown to Augustus III the Saxon (in 1734) as a consequence of a Russian intervention (likewise military). Through the diplomatic and military efforts of his son-in-law, King Louis XV of France, he was installed as Duke of Loraine and Bar for the remainder of his life (1736–1766).

[17]   Charles XII (1682–1718), King of Sweden (from 1697).

country; how, when he was called back again to the throne, an adverse faction, supported by foreigners, rendered the efforts and hopes of the soundest part of the nation useless and vain. The dangers are known to which he was exposed; the disguises he was obliged to employ to escape from his enemies.[18] It is known, that, at last, peace having secured him in the tranquil possession of the dukedoms of Lorraine and Bar, he carefully employed himself to make those people lose the remembrance of their ancient masters. Need I tell here all that he did for that purpose? I will only say, that his buildings at Nancy and Lunéville appeared to me far superior to all that I had seen in many other courts.

At our arrival, this monarch received us with that bounty and affability which gained him every heart; and, being of his country, we were, by his order, lodged in his palace.

With this prince lived the famous Bébé, till then considered as the most extraordinary dwarf that ever was seen;[19] who was, indeed, of a perfectly proportioned shape, with very pleasing features, but who (I am sorry to say it, for the honour of my species) had, both in his mind and way of thinking, all the defects commonly attributed to us. He was at that time about thirty, his height two feet eight inches; and when measured, it appeared that I was much shorter, being no more than two feet four inches.

At our first interview he shewed much fondness and friendship towards me; but when he perceived that I preferred the company and conversations of sensible people to his own, and above all, when he saw that the King took pleasure in my company, he conceived against me the most violent jealousy and hatred; so that, had it not been for a kind of miracle, I could not have escaped his fury.

One day we were both in the apartment of his Majesty. This Prince, having much caressed me, and asked several questions to which I gave satisfactory

---

[18]   During the war over the Polish crown (1733–1734), Leszczyński had managed to flee the city of Gdańsk (Danzig), besieged by Russian troops, while disguised as a peasant. The event later became the stuff of legend and was repeatedly invoked in Polish literature and painting (such as in a well-known engraving by Daniel Chodowiecki).

[19]   Nicolas Ferry, the Alsatian dwarf known as Bébé (1741–1764), was only 18 years old at the time of their meeting (in 1759), not 30 as Boruwłaski suggests. This error may be explained by the fact – mentioned by witnesses from the epoch (such as the Count de Tressan) – that Bébé began to age very early and gave the impression of being an old man upon his death at 23.

answers, seemed pleased with my replies, and testified his pleasure and approbation in the most affectionate manner; then addressing Bébé, said to him:

'You see, Bébé, what a difference there is between Joujou and you! He is amiable, cheerful, entertaining, and full of knowledge, whereas you are but a little machine.'

At these words, I saw fury sparkle in his eyes. He answered nothing, but his countenance and blush proved enough that he was violently agitated. A moment after, the King being gone to his closet, Bébé availed himself of that instant to execute his revengeful projects; and slily approaching, seized me by the waist, and endeavoured to push me into the fire. Luckily I laid hold with both hands of an iron hook, by which, in chimneys, the shovels and tongs are kept upright, and thus I prevented his wicked design. The noise I made in defending myself, brought back the King, who came to my assistance, and saved me from that imminent danger. He afterwards called for his servants, put Bébé in their hands, bade them inflict on him a corporal punishment proportioned to his fault, and ordered him never to appear in his presence any more.

In vain did I intercede in behalf of the unhappy Bébé, I could not save him the first part of his sentence; and as for the other, his Majesty did not consent to revoke it but upon condition he should beg my pardon. Bébé with much reluctance, submitted to this humiliation, which very likely made on him a deeper impression. In effect, he fell sick a short time after, and died. Everybody attributed his death to his jealousy, and to the vexation which the difference, that was said to be between us, had given to him.[20] I sincerely pitied him, and would not have related this circumstance, but to remark, that the smallness of our stature does not prevent us from experiencing the power of the passions. Happily for me, when I have been the sport of them, they never inspired me with any thing contrary to humanity and the laws.

It was during my stay at Lunéville, that I had honour to cultivate an acquaintance with the celebrated Count de Tressan,[21] who was come to reside

---

[20]   Although Bébé was indeed not very intellectually well endowed and is said to have had a problematic character, he died not of jealousy but most likely of an infection that attacked his weakened body – at least according to the Count de Tressan.

[21]   Louis Elisabeth de la Vergne, Count de Tressan (1705–1783), a French writer, Grand Marshal at the court of Stanisław Leszczyński, member of the French Academy of Sciences.

there a little while. He took much notice of me, and the article *Nain* in the *Encyclopédie*, with an advantageous mention of me, was by him.[22]

After having considered and admired all that King Stanislaus has done to embellish Nancy and Lunéville, we took leave of this good Prince, who gave my benefactress letters for the late Queen of France, his daughter,[23] and repaired to Paris.

I need not say, that the first care of the Countess Humieska was to go to Versailles, where, as a Polander, she easily got admittance to the Queen, to whom she delivered the letters which the King her father had honoured her with. This Princess, who had preserved much affection for every thing belonging to her own country, received her Ladyship most graciously. Her Majesty being informed that my benefactress had me with her, wished to see me, was astonished at my appearance, the smallness of which she had no idea of; and after having asked me many questions concerning the King her father, Bébé, Poland, and our travels, she seemed pleased with my answers, and did me so much honour as to add, that I was a little prodigy; that, upon what she had seen or ever been told, she till then deemed the individuals of my species as ill-favoured by nature, as much in mind and intellectual faculties as in body, but that I undeceived her in a very advantageous and pleasing manner.

After these obliging words, the Queen, addressing the Countess Humieska, was so kind as to engage her to repeat her visit often, desiring she would bring me with her, and gave orders to admit us whenever we desired it.

On our return to Paris, the curiosity I excited drew many visitors to my protectress; and in less than a week, every person of high rank at court, every person of fashion in town waited upon her. I could not help, indeed, being infinitely flattered by that kind of enthusiasm, and the numberless civilities I was honoured with. The late Duke d'Orleans,[24] specially, having given my protectress

---

[22]   *Encyclopédie ou dictionnaire raisonné des sciences, des arts et des métiers*, the collective work compiled by Denis Diderot and Jean le Rond d`Alembert, the most famous encyclopaedia of the Enlightenment era (published in 1751–1780). The entry for dwarf (*le nain*), which profiled Boruwłaski in detail and was carried in volume 11 (Neuchâtel, 1765, pp. 5–7), was in fact authored by Chevalier Louis de Jaucourt, but he did base it largely on a report prepared by the Count de Tressan for the French Academy in 1759.

[23]   Maria Leszczyńska (1703–1768), daughter of Stanisław and Catherine Opalińska, who became wife of King Louis XV (from 1725) and Queen of France.

[24]   Louis Philippe, Duke of Orléans (1725–1785).

the most elegant entertainments, was in particular very fond of me, and loaded me with caresses and presents. I can even say, that, during our stay at Paris, this amiable Prince did not pass a single day without giving us new testimonies of his politeness.

I should be deficient towards the Count Oginski, Grand General of Lithuania,[25] who at that time lived in Paris, if I forgot to mention the particular regard he shewed to me. His Lordship, who came constantly to pay his visits to my protectress, made much of me, and carried his complaisance so far as to teach me the first principles of music; an art, in which, as a man of rank, he had made a very astonishing progress. On seeing that I was intent upon it, and imagining I had a taste for it, he engaged my benefactress to give me for a master the celebrated Gavinies,[26] who taught me to play on the guitar; a talent which often solaces me in moments of trouble and inquietude, inseparable from a situation like mine. But to return to the Count Oginski: this nobleman took pleasure in having me near him; and I remember one day when he gave a grand banquet to several of the most distinguished ladies, he put me in an urn placed on the middle of the table; and the curiosity of this company being much excited, both by his saying he wished to regale them with an extraordinary mess, and by excusing himself for some time from uncovering the urn which he seemed to rate so high. I occasioned, by my sudden appearance, an uncommon roar and surprise on the ladies not knowing me at first.

The ecstasy I excited, with all that was related about my figure, repartees, and understanding, gave rise to an incident, which, had not the Queen interposed, might have had disagreeable consequences for the Polish ladies who travel in France.

It had happened by chance, that the Duchess of Modena, a Princess of the royal blood of France,[27] had not been at any of the entertainments to which I had been invited. However, her Grace had heard much of me, and all that she

---

[25]　Michał Kazimierz Ogiński (1728–1800) was not yet Grand Hetman in the period described by Boruwłaski (he attained the title in 1768); he was a musician and composer, the author of the entry for 'harp' in the Encyclopédie.

[26]　Pierre Gavinies (1728–1800), a French violinist and composer, one of the most famous and most outstanding virtuosos of his time.

[27]　Charlotte Aglaé d'Orléans (1700–1761), from 1720 wife of Francesco III d'Este, Duke of Modena.

had been told gave her a strong desire of seeing me. Her rank not permitting her to pay the first visit to the Countess Humieska, she determined to write to her, and as I was the principal person she desired to see, she added to the card, "Especially, do not forget to bring Joujou".

The Countess Humieska, who possesses all the sentiments correspondent to her illustrious birth; and whose rank, beauty, and wealth had drawn on her everywhere the most flattering distinctions, was greatly offended at such an invitation; and not thinking proper to gratify a curiosity disclosed in so aukward and uncomplaisant a manner, answered, she was very sorry she could not comply with her Grace's commands; she was engaged on that day and the following, so she could not say when she might have that honour.

The Duchess of Modena, who understood perfectly well the meaning of this answer, was very much incensed, and spoke and complained of it to every one she met. She even went so far as to carry her complaints to the Queen, imagining that her Majesty, being a Polander, would blame my benefactress for it.

I could almost believe that the Queen, who had a great regard for the persons of her own nation, inwardly thought that the Countess Humieska was right. However, wishing to settle a trifle, which, though slight in its principle, might terminate in causing some uneasiness to my benefactress, she sent for her, and engaged her to pay a visit to the Duchess of Modena. The Countess answered, that through respect for her Majesty's orders, she would go, but certainly would not take Joujou thither; upon which the Queen, foreseeing that such a visit might only widen the breach, dropped the conversations, and, at the end of the visit, invited the Countess Humieska to come and breakfast with her Majesty two days after, bringing me with her. She sent afterwards another invitation to the Duchess of Modena for the same day, without making known to either of these ladies that they were to meet one another.

On the appointed day we waited upon the Queen, and arrived first. But what a surprise for us, when some minutes after we heard the name of the Duchess of Modena announced! This lady, no less astonished than we, came, however, to herself very soon; and, after she had paid her duty to the Queen, the two ladies saluted each other with the usual compliments; and, as if nothing had happened, reciprocally declared the pleasure they had to see, and the desire they had had to know one another. The Duchess even went so far as not to take notice of me for some minutes; but soon banishing this constraint, her caresses, praises, and eagerness proved how great her enthusiasm was.

After this adventure, which shows in what character I acted at Paris, and put me quite in fashion, we continued to be visited and entertained by every one of the most considerable amongst the nobility and financiers. Mr. Bouret[28] especially, the Farmer General, so much renowned for his ambition, excesses and extravagancies, gave an entertainment, in which, to show that it was for my sake, he caused every thing, even the plate, the spoons, knives and forks, to be proportioned to my size, and the dishes, consisting of ortolans, becaficos and other small game of this kind, to be served up on dishes adapted to them. It was about this time that I got acquainted with the celebrated Demoiselle Clairon,[29] who has since rendered me the greatest services.

We spent in this manner more than a year at Paris, in all the pleasures which the capital offers to foreigners, and the lively humour, the cheerfulness an politeness of its inhabitants, render still more sprightly. The time at length came, when we were to leave that place, from whence we set off for Holland.

Everybody knows how the soul of a traveller is impressed by the novelty of the scenes which this country affords. It was then the month of May, a season in which it presents the most agreeable appearance; and I was struck with it in so lively a manner, that notwithstanding the sameness so justly complained of, I cannot recall to my mind without emotion, the sensations I then felt. It would be repeating what has been said a thousand times, if I undertook to describe it. I will then confine myself to say, that when we arrived at the Hague, this astonishing village, which may vie with cities of the first rank, the Countess Humieska was received in the most affable and polite manner by his Highness the Prince Stadtholder[30] and his family, who did their utmost to make her stay agreeable. We, however, made but few acquaintance there; and not being able

---

[28] Etienne Michel Bouret (1709–1777), French financier, serving as tax collector general from 1747.

[29] Mlle. Clairon, real name Josephe Hippolyte Claire de la Tude (1723–1803), a famous French actress appearing with the Comédie Française, highly fashionable among the Enlightenment-age elite (admired by Voltaire and the encyclopaedists). She was at the peak of her popularity in 1743–1766.

[30] Wilhelm V, Prince of Orange, (1748–1806), Statholder of the Dutch Republic (1751–1795), was only 13 years old when Humiecka and Boruwłaski arrived in 1761, and the republic was governed by Ludwig Ernst von Braunschweig as regent.

to stay long in Holland, we employed ourselves in viewing the curiosities with which this country abounds; and at last, after having taken leave of Stadtholder, my benefactress took her route through Germany, and we reached Warsaw.

My return to my native country made much noise. I had not yet been seen in the capital, but was preceded by the reputation I had acquired in my travels, and for which I was indebted to the generous care of my benefactress. Besides, I had improved during my stay in foreign countries; and, as Paris had given me somewhat of that easy politeness which graces manners, and enhances the lightest prattle, I was so happy as to perceive that many persons, by whom at first I was looked upon only as an object of mere curiosity, sought my society, because they took pleasure in my conversation. Emboldened by this notice, I went oftener to enlarge the circle of my acquaintance, I cultivated an intimacy with several young gentlemen of my age, whose company seemed to me more gay and interesting than those who habitually frequented the Countess Humieska's house.

I had inspired my protectress with confidence enough to allow me a reasonable liberty, of which I availed myself to go frequently to the play. I had always been very fond of it, but now new sensations, which began to rise in me, increased its worth. No longer did I repair thither to admire the fineness of the play, or the art of the performers. The show itself attracted me, the concourse of spectators, but women above all, who stirring up in some kind of new emotions, made me attend the Theatre with a degree of frenzy. Till then I had lived almost without conceiving any difference between the sexes; but from the inquietude, the agitation, and the trouble which the preference of a woman caused in me, I could no longer conceal to myself, that on this enchanting sex depends all our happiness; yet was I not able to define in what and how it might be promoted.

The Theatre was also the general rendezvous of my young friends. They had all the indiscretion of their age, and indulged without scruple the impulse of their brisk and sprightly imagination. By incessantly talking of their pleasures past, or in project, it was not long before they supplied me with the knowledge I wanted, and gave a fixed bias to desires, till then confused and incoherent. Women, besides, by their continual railleries at the shortness of my stature, their pleasantries on my reservedness and circumspection, completely cured me of that timidity, which seemed, as it were, ascribed to my size. My head being filled with the idea of them, my heart strongly agitated by the change lately operated in me, I viewed the objects under aspects more lively and interesting; I wished to love, I did so already. Women, in my eyes, had taken quite a new form. They excited my admiration, my sensibility, my desires; but it was sufficient to be a woman, that title gave her a right to my rising passion: I was fond of the sex, without choice or distinction, I loved them all; in a word, at the age of twenty-five I was like other young lads at fifteen.

These emotions, quite new to me, had their charms; and, perhaps, I had been happier, if I could have been contented with experiencing them, without seeking how to gratify desires which every day grew more pressing. Unhappily, such a resistance is not in nature of man; pressed by the warmth of my constitution, I wished to fix my views upon a particular object. How much was my mind mortified on reflecting upon my stature, which I considered as an insurmountable obstacle to the happiness I longed for with so much ardour!

'What?!' said I to myself, 'the most reserved women take me upon their lap! They embrace me, they bestow upon me the most tender caresses, they use me like a child! How can I hazard, in such circumstances, a declaration at which they will only laugh, whilst I shall remain covered with eternal ridicule?'

It was not an easy matter to make my pride agree with my desires. The farther I was from having the common size of other men, the more lively I wished that difference might be forgotten, and that I might be treated like them. But experience has taught me that I thought as a child. I was ignorant of the effect such wonderful things may produce: above all I knew not, forgive me, ye fair! how far women might be led by curiosity. I soon knew it.

There was then at Warsaw amongst the French comedians, an actress, highly distinguished for the talents in the character of a waiting-maid. A certain mixture of tenderness and vivacity rendered her infinitely interesting; and though not regularly handsome, yet she possessed all that was requisite to please and seduce. I always saw her with new pleasure, and openly preferred her to all others. One night, when she had made on a most particular impression, on going out of the playhouse, I met one of my friends, to whom, intending some relaxation, I proposed a walk. He desired me to excuse him, and confessed that he was going to sup at the little ***, precisely the same actress.

'Ah!' exclaimed I with emotion, 'are you acquainted with her? How happy are you!'

'So may you be, when you please,' answered my giddy young spark. 'I will introduce you to her, as my friend, and you may be sure to be well received.'

This offer I accepted with transport, and the very next day I was introduced, and welcomed in a manner equal to what I had been made to hope. This visit passed away merrily, and when I retired, she most earnestly invited me often to repeat it.

With what eagerness did I avail myself of this invitation! How long the moments seemed which were to bring that of seeing her! With what regret did I see those fly away which I spent with her! I was bold enough to declare my passion for her; she seemed to partake of it, and for a while my illusion made me happy. Pleased, nay, intoxicated with this amour, I avoided my young friends, wanted to enjoy within myself my imaginary felicity, devoted to my young mistress all the moments I could steal from the decency and duty imposed upon my benefactress. Let these details be forgiven me; in writing these memoirs, I not only mean to describe my size and its proportions, I would likewise follow the unfolding of my sentiments, the affections of my soul. I would speak openly, rather tell what I felt than what I did, and demonstrate that, if I can upbraid nature with having refused me a body like that of other men, she has made me ample amends, by endowing me with a sensibility, which, it is true, displayed itself rather late, but, even in my wantonness, spread a teint of happiness, the remembrance of which I enjoy with gratitude and feeling heart.

But to return to my charmer, the Abigail: our connection did not last long. I was sincere in my attachment, and imagining myself beloved, she made me happy. Therefore how great must be my astonishment, when one day on meeting by chance the very same young man who had introduced me to her, I was told that my little intrigue was known to everybody, and spoken of publickly; that they bantered my discretion; and she, whom I thought the most interested in secrecy, did not scruple openly to laugh at my passion and eagerness, at the tumultuous emotions she had excited in me; that she even gloried in it, and produced as no small proof of her merit, to have provoked in a man of my size a manner of being apparently so little suitable to him. This discovery sunk me down, by humbling my pride. I thought I loved sincerely, I had hoped to be sincerely beloved; and it was not without extreme grief I saw the veil fall, and my illusion dispelled.

Divers circumstances still increased my grief. I had been very cautious lest my benefactress, or any of the sensible persons who were interested in my concerns, should have the least suspicion of my intrigue. To do this, I was obliged, in order to make my little excursions when everybody thought me asleep, to bribe the doorkeeper, to gain the servant who accompanied me. But what regret did I suffer, when, on being discovered, I saw both the door-keeper and my servant turned away! When I had to reproach myself with being the cause that they lost their places, with being, perhaps, the instrument of their misfortune! My benefactress sent to me a very grave, wise and sensible man, in whom I had the greatest confidence; he strongly remonstrated to me on the irregularity of my behaviour, and set forth the fatal consequences into which I was likely to be hurried away. His reflections affected me; I promised never more to frequent the young men whose discourses and bad example had seduced me; and, by the regularity of my conduct, I soon regained the kindness of the Countess Humieska, and of her society.

I had no occasion to repent it. My life was more quiet and happy. The effervescence of a juvenile constitution had procured me some pleasures; but it was not long before I felt the vacuum they left behind them. I then began to perceive that sentiment, reciprocal sentiment only, can give animation and liveliness to pleasures, which without it are nought. I began to comprehend that esteem and confidence only can give birth to a permanent love. In the friendship and conversation of wise persons I sought after a compensation, and easily found it.

At that time Warsaw was the scene of rejoicings and amusement. Stanislaus II.[31] had lately ascended the throne of Poland; and this Prince, on whose virtues and accomplishments I need not expatiate, as they are known to all those who had the honour to approach him either as a king or a private man, as applying himself to retrieve those innumerable calamities which a series of troubles and agitations had occasioned.[32] By his patronage, the arts and sciences were flourishing; he

---

[31]   This is how Stanisław Augustus Poniatowski (1732–1798), who ascended the Polish throne in 1764, was known in Europe.

[32]   The *Memoirs* were written in 1788 after the rebellion against Poniatowski and Russian troops in Poland (The Bar Confederation, 1768–1772) and after first partition of Poland (1772).

gained the affections of his greatest lords, who flocked round his person, and who, to evince their attachment, vied with each other in giving the most splendid entertainments. At one of these festivals, in which my benefactress was reckoned one of the chief ornaments, I had the honour to be presented to his Majesty, who condescended to take the strongest notice of me, and from that time bestowed upon me the most unequivocal proofs of it, and even to this day ceases not to honour me with a peculiar protection.

In this state of tranquillity my days glided away, and I thought that no kind of vexation could trouble so happy of life. I was then very far from foreseeing that this delicate and tender sentiment upon which was grounded my expectation of a future felicity, should one day be the cause of disquietude and bitterness of heart, and would so powerfully overwhelm my existence. But before I enter into the particulars of these events, which I shall always behold as the most interesting of my life, I beg leave to acquaint my reader with some circumstances which belong to the history of my sister, whose death I heard of nearly at this epoch.

Anastasia Boruwlaska was seven years younger than I, and of so short a stature that she could exactly stand under my arm; but this can be no matter of astonishment, when what I said before is remembered, that she was only two feet two inches high at the time of her death. Astonishing as she was, for the shortness of her person, and the extreme regular proportions of her shape, with which the nicest sculptor could not have found fault, she was still more so by the qualities of her heart, and the gentleness of her disposition. She was of a brown complexion, with fine black eyes, well circled eyebrows, very thick hair, and so much gracefulness in all she did, that added new charms to her figure. Her temper was lively and cheerful; her heart, feeling and beneficent. She could not see a suffering fellow-creature, without seeking to give relief. The Castellane Kaminska,[33] a very rich lady, was both a friend and a protectress of her. She had taken her to her house, expressed for her an unbounded tenderness, refuse her nothing; and the little Anastasia availed herself of that ascendancy to gratify her own heart, which incited her to generosity.

---

[33]   Katarzyna Kossakowska née Potocka (1722–1803), the wife of Castellan of Kamień Stanisław Kossakowski, a very politically active lady famous for her sharp tongue.

My sister, like me, had been so happy as to feel those tender affections which diffuse so many charms over our lives, and the sweetness of which does so well counterpoise the troubles, the inquietudes and contradictions which they make us suffer. At twenty, Anastasia was in love, and with so much the more passion, that her attachment was grounded upon the only pleasure of contributing to the happiness of him who was the object of it. She had neither fears, nor sorrows, nor remorses to endure; and thus she might have lived happy, had not jealousy overpowered her, and too often troubled her repose. It was not difficult for her benefactress to perceive her inclination: she mentioned it to her; and this ingenuous, tender and feeling heart did not conceal the sentiments which a young officer of a very handsome shape and fine figure, who frequented the house, had inspired her with. This young gentleman, though of a good family, was not rich; Anastasia knew it, and endeavouring to find the means of serving him without hurting his delicacy. She contrived to engage him to play at piquet[34] with her; and generally obliging him to play deep, she contrived always to lose, and thus joined the pleasure of doing him good, to that of avoiding his expressions of gratitude. I know not how far my sister's sensibility would have carried her, if during the excursion to Leopold she had not been seized with the small-pox. Unfortunately for me, and for her friends, the disorder was without remedy. Recourse was had in vain to all the helps of the medical art; and within two days she died, with the same tranquillity of soul, the same calmness of mind, nay, the same philosophy with which she had lived. I cannot recollect this sad event without shedding tears for the loss of a sister, and of a friend. Her benefactress was inconsolable, and during many days her wealth was in danger. She gave the strictest orders that nobody should ever speak to her of her dear Anastasia; even desired me not to come to see her, lest my presence should open again deep wounds too difficult to be healed. Thus I had not the satisfaction to mingle my tears with hers, and to shew her my warm, though insufficient, gratitude for all that she had done to her young and little friend.

Other cares and anxieties soon succeeded those which this loss had caused me. I come now to the most interesting epoch of my life, those moments, which, being fraught with new ideas, new desires, pleasures far different from those I had known, brought likewise new troubles and new difficulties to which I

---

[34] A card game for two players using a 32-card deck (from sevens up to aces).

never thought I should be exposed. The Countess Humieska's bounty seemed for ever to secure me from want. As her ladyship's favour had drawn on me the consideration and regard not only of every person in her house, but even of all the quality that composed her society, I did not foresee, nor did I find in my heart the fear of ever becoming unworthy of her regard. I was caressed, fondled, and cherished; nothing was wanting to my happiness; and I enjoyed it with so much the more security, that not knowing reverses, I foolishly thought never to endure any. On the other side, reason and good counsels having brought me back to more quiet sentiments, I thought those tumultuous passions, which for a while had so vehemently agitated me, were for ever calmed. I imagined that, by confining my affections to marks of gratitude towards so many persons who liberally bestowed their kindness upon me, I should lead a peaceful life; and that, reclaimed from love and its chimeras, my renouncing it for ever would make me amends for the pains it had occasioned me. But I knew not my own heart; and these fine resolutions vanished, when I saw a young person whom my benefactress had lately taken into her house as a lady in waiting, or companion.

Isalina Barboutan[35] was descended from French parents, long settled in Warsaw, where they enjoyed a happy mediocrity. 'T is a custom in Poland for the Lords, as well as Ladies of quality, to take young persons of good birth, who are brought up at their own charge, and afterwards provided for, either by admitting them into their household, giving them in marriage, or procuring them civil or military employments. This ancient usage has its origin in the wide disproportion of fortunes amongst the nobility. According to the constitution of the country, all nobleman may aspire to the crown, which is elective; so that the richest of them attach to themselves a vast number of creatures, who upon occasion may support their pretensions.[36]

Be that as it may, my benefactress had only consulted her own heart, when she took Isalina; and this young lady possessed all the requisites to interest and

---

[35]   Isalina (or Isaline) Barboutan (1762–1852), born to a French family settled in Warsaw, married Boruwłaski in 1779.

[36]   The phenomenon of clientism was very widespread among the Polish szlachta and magnates, but Boruwłaski goes too far here in claiming that it was motivated by the royal aspirations of powerful lords. A desire to pull together a strong political powerbase was indeed an important factor, but with the goal of influencing local political intrigues, not of attaining the throne. Besides, this custom had little to do with the case of Isalina, who was simply one of Humiecka's lady courtiers.

please her. Let me be excused from describing what she appeared in my eyes, her modesty would not suffer it; and besides, such as regard only the figure in the choice of their consorts, know very little of the human heart. To live together, to have for each other that mutual esteem which alone can make us happy, more lasting qualities are requisite. Being now a father, having found in my wife a sincere friend, who partakes of my pains and pleasures, a fond mother who only delights in educating her children, I know how to set a proper value on those advantages so much sought after, thought they only are gifts which nature blindly distributes. Yet I must own, there is a personal beauty which discloses that of the soul; and when we meet with such tender, sweet and lively countenances, which, being strangers to dissimulation and deceit, exhibit in their features the motions they feel, the impressions they receive, we must acknowledge, at the very first moment, that persons so happily endowed are worthy of all our attachment. 'T is among women especially that this inestimable quality is to be found, which sets off their charms so advantageously: they possess it, notwithstanding all the obstacles that opposed to it, though the aim of their education incessantly be to instruct them how to dissemble their sentiments, and conceal their natural affections. May I have resolution and wisdom enough to overcome this prejudice in training up my children! But I see the evil, and know not the remedy, or rather have not courage enough to use it.

It was, however, young Isalina's beauty, her sparkling eyes, the elegance of her shape which struck me at first sight, and subdued my heart. But if from that moment the impression was deep and indelible, what a new force did my sentiments receive, when living in the same house, and having every day opportunities to see her, I could freely admire her sweet and insinuating voice, her lively and cheerful conversation, her easy and noble carriage; when I discovered in her a smart and brilliant wit, an inexhaustible stock of gaiety, a gracefulness that embellished her whole person, and that native meekness which was the plain index of a feeling heart! From this time my happiness was affixed to her fate; without fear I discovered in me all the symptoms of a violent passion; and though I foresaw the numberless obstacles I had to overcome, yet I did not give up my enterprise, and hoped that by dint of perseverance and attention they should be at last surmounted.

How different is this passion from the tumultuous sensations which had before disturbed me! I was in love, but a love accompanied with that respect and diffidence which are inseparable from a true passion. My only desire was to spend my life with the object that caused it; and whereas formerly I had been determined only by the allurements of pleasure and personal satisfaction, which, leaving the heart empty, and bringing distaste, flatters our pride but faintly, I felt that the end at which I truly aimed, was the happiness of the person to whom I was attached; and that, if I could succeed to make her happy, there would not be anything wanting to my own felicity.

I had everyday new occasions of applauding myself for my sentiments. My benefactress, charmed at the qualities she discovered in her young favourite, had her education carefully finished, and took a most particular liking and interest in her behalf. Living under the same roof, and seeing her every day with that sweet familiarity which my size, her youth and innocence seemed to authorize, I did not lose a single opportunity of approaching her; I had no other delight than to see and admire, to love her secretly. Much time passed before I could resolve to acquaint her with my sentiments. Every day I formed this resolution; but every day the reflections of my mind discovered obstacles that were more and more invincible, and my speech expired ere it reached my lips. Whilst I suffered every lady to take me on her lap, and submitted to their fondness and caresses, I was anxiously cautious lest Isalina should do the same; I shunned her notice, either with a serious look, or by stealing away from her. She often complained of being the only one I loved not; but how little did she know the inmost dealings of my heart! When I would have given my life to enjoy a single one of her caresses as a friend, I scorned to receive all those she would lavish on me as a child. Nay, by humbling my pride to the utmost, they ended with causing in me so real and violent a pain, that I cannot describe it. It was then I bitterly felt all the disadvantages of my size. Then all the praises I was loaded with on every other side, could not make me amends for the inconveniences I found myself liable to. It was then I considered it as the sole obstacle to the only good that could attach me to life: to be upon a level with other men, I would have sacrificed both the fondness of my benefactress, and the bounty, even I will say, the consideration with which the King and the Nobles of his court vouchsafed to honour me.

It was not only the fear of becoming unacceptable to Isalina that dejected my mind. I apprehended that, should I succeeded in winning her affection, could I engage her to lay aside prejudices, and be resolved concerning the union of her fate to mine, there would still remain many difficulties to overcome, either to gain her parents' consent, without which there was no hope left for me, or to obtain the sanction of my benefactress, who undoubtedly would think this marriage ridiculous, and by all means oppose it. This last was not the least powerful obstacle. Besides my being bound to the Countess Humieska by sentiments of the most tender respect and heartfelt gratitude, I had no fortune, I was totally indebted to her beneficence for my easy circumstances, I did not subsist but through her bounty. I had, therefore, to fear lest I should lose it by marrying against her will. I had reason to be afraid of involving in my misfortunes a young person, who, though without fortune herself, had by her youth, education, figure, and, above all, by the protection of our common benefactress, a right to an advantageous match.

These reflections did not all occur to my mind at first. During more than one year I had been fully taken up with the delight of loving and daily seeing the object of my affections; but at length, when I was come to that point so natural, wherein to speak of our love is irresistibly necessary, they crowded in my imagination, and filled me with anguish and melancholy. They indeed ought to have made me give up my passion; but do we reason when in love? My health became visibly impaired; I was uneasy and anxious beyond conception; in short, so violent was my situation, that not being able to remain in this cruel uncertainty, I determined on declaring my passion, and waited only for favourable opportunity, which soon presented itself.

One evening when I had been more sad and dejected than usual, chance, or rather the attraction that kept me fast to Isalina, made me stay the last in the drawing-room. I then formed the resolution of opening my heart to her, which gave me such a look of trouble and perplexity, that she could not help being struck with.

'Pray what is the matter Joujou?' said she to me, with the most striking look of concern and pity. 'What is the sorrow you are consumed by, and so artfully conceal? Is there nobody to whom you can trust enough to pour out your heart? You act unkindly with your friends.'

'And comes this reproach from you,' answered I with warmth 'from you, the only cause of all my grief?'

I wished to go on, but sobs stifled my speech, and letting my head fall upon her lap, I could only lisp the words love – passion – misfortune, and wept bitterly.

At first, Isalina's heart startled at the pitiful state she saw me in; but soon recovering from her surprise, she only found the scene ridiculous.

'Indeed, Joujou' said she 'you are a child, and I cannot but laugh at your extravagance. Did I ever forbid you to love me? On the contrary, did I not always upbraid you for your indifference to me?'

I did not expect such an answer, I own; it humbled me. I had much ado to make her understand that I did not love her as a child, and would not be loved like a child. At this she burst into laughter, told me I knew not what I said, and left the apartment.

More content with having made my declaration, than minding the manner it had been received, I wholly gave myself over to the pleasure of knowing that the object of my fondness was apprised of the passion she had caused me to breathe. I said to myself, that now she might easily interpret my melancholy, my grief, and my reservedness towards her; that she could not but attribute them to a strong and deep sentiment. I ventured to hope, that this sentiment would speak in my behalf, and plead my cause to a delicate and feeling heart. But the succeeding days plainly shewed that I was mistaken. She incessantly bantered me; and indulging herself in the gaiety of her imagination, the more I endeavoured to display my sentiments, and to speak to her as a man, the more she delighted in ridiculing them, and treated me like a child. She asked me – whether I imagined her like my young actress? How many days longer would my sentiments last? I could not return any answer; I left her, wept, and inveighed against her injustice, and my misfortune.

Unable any longer to resist the heavy melancholy that had seized me through such usage, my strength failed me, and I fell dangerously ill. I kept my room more than two months, without any other comfort, than that she sometimes inquired after my situation. I impatiently waited till the physician would give me leave to go out. As soon as this happy moment arrived, I seized the first opportunity of speaking to her in private, and told her, that she alone had been the cause of my illness. She assured me she had been very much concerned at it;

and that if I had listened more to reason, if I had loved her as she thought she had merited, I might have spared her this trouble. She promised me, since I was so much affected at it, no more to banter me upon my love; yet she hoped that, for my part, I would strive to entertain more calm sentiments towards her.

With what salutary balm did this speech sooth my heart! The tender concern with which it was uttered, made me happy. From that time I thought I had in some measure impressed the generous soul of Isalina; and how could I have failed? I loved so earnestly, and love had rendered me so unhappy, that she must needs have been ungrateful not to be affected by it.

Not having it in my power to see her alone as often as I wished, perceiving that even she by all means avoided me, I resolved to write to her. May I beg leave to insert this correspondence, which, as it has determined my doom, is therefore infinitely precious to me.

Joujou to Isalina.
October, 10th, 1779

The secret of my heart has then escaped me! She who is the object of my love knows at last the sentiments of it, may she know them as they are felt! She would then become more tender to me, would see she has no other alternative, than to consummate my happiness, or to cause and effect my death. O, dearest friend! Oh! that Nature had doomed me, by my stature, never to pass the narrow circle of childhood! Why then have given me a feeling heart, allotted me a soul capable of appreciating the qualities of your own, implanted in my bosom the seeds of a violent passion? Why not have proportioned my affections to the narrow compass of my frame? Having prolonged my infancy till my twentieth year, why not have kept me therein for ever? By liberally bestowing on me what she allows to others as a gift of Heaven, had she in view my torment and misery? She is not a step mother; she cannot be so cruel only to me.

What would I venture to say more? You fly me, you shun me, you endeavour to keep from my fight. Is it thus you take pity on me? Is this the tender mercy you seemed to grant me? You have permitted me to name you my friend, and you refuse me the sentiments of friendship! Can you so cruelly reject those of the tender and unhappy

Joujou?

Joujou to Isalina.

Oct. 17, ten at night.

Cruel friend, what torments do you make me endure! What! eight full days have elapsed, and you have not deigned to answer me! Would it have been too hard for you to return me one line, to venture a single word by which the unhappy Joujou might be comforted? He breathes for you the tenderest sentiments, bears the most attentive reverence; and you take no notice of his sacrifices, of the privations he lays down to himself! Nay, you affect to fly from him. With what cruelty did you leave the assembly this very evening, because, had you stayed, you could not have helped keeping the only empty seat, which by chance was next to mine? Ah! dear friend, may you never experience torture like mine! And, oh, I pray, make mine cease; let the tender and feeling Isalina cause no longer the misfortune of him whom she formerly called her dear

Joujou!

Isalina to Joujou.

October 19th.

Cease, Joujou, do cease to pursue me; be no longer unjust. Your passion vexes, your grief touches me; the one you carry too far; to the other you yield too much. Love me, I consent; I will also love you, and as much as you please; but that is all. Consider a little, and you will see that I cannot do more. Why these transports? Your exalted imagination hinders you from seeing the objects such as they are, such as they ought to be. Prevents you, above all from appreciating the tender concern, the sincere friendship which are devoted to you by your

Isalina.

Joujou to Isalina.

Oct. 21st, eleven at night.

Where shall I find words, my charming friend, sufficient to express all that your billet has made me feel? You give me leave to love you, and promise a return. Ah! let me incessantly hear these sweet words which are still echoed to the bottom of my heart! But why your sad and cruel reflections? You forbid my transports!.. are you sure it is in my power to obey you? No matter, I will do my endeavours; I will try to reason with you; and perhaps it will not be so difficult as you seem to imagine, to demonstrate that, upon the whole, our reciprocal happiness requires of us to pass beyond the bounds it seems you desire to impose upon me.

Yes, charming friend, the more I have reflected, and the more I meditate upon our situation, the less I can see by what our sentiments must be checked or limbed. I do not conceal to myself the innumerable obstacles which oppose our happiness; but cannot love surmount them all? I know very well, that, generally speaking, a young person may fear to fall into ridicule by uniting herself to a man of my stature; and this ridicule seems so much the more to be feared, that it may influence your sentiments. Besides, the same prejudice will necessarily determine both your parents and my benefactress to oppose such an union. In fine, we have no fortune; and this sad predicament, by keeping us dependent, seems to deprive us of an hope to be ever happy.

Still, my charming friend, permit me to communicate to you the divers observations which our situation presents to my mind. For these fifteen months I have been taken up with these considerations, and having time to meditate upon them, I will freely say to you what I think. Undoubtedly, my dear Isalina, our marriage would furnish matter for conversation; and though commonly the talk of one day hardly reaches the next, yet we, perchance, may be spoken of a whole fortnight. But how could you be blamed or ridiculed, not actuated by ambition or desire or enjoying a large fortune? The wise, and even the wicked must be forced to own, that you had no other motive than a profound sentiment, a strong friendship, a sincere desire of making me happy. Would not all these considerations commend your heart? Far from blaming your conduct, would not every one deem it noble and generous, and, on the least reflection, would the joke be converted into admiration?

It is very true, that, at first sight, the idea of marrying a man of my stature will appear somewhat ludicrous; but, my charming friend, are you not already familiarized with this idea? Did you not repeat to me more than once, that my society had become agreeable to you? Besides, if I love you better than any other man could do; if, sensible of the obligations I shall be under, on feeling my own inferiority, I strive to make you amends by the greatest attentions and cares, would you not be happier than with an imperious husband, who, not knowing how to value you, even ignorant of what love is, would make you sink under the yoke of marriage, and not taste its sweets? Confess, my dearest friend, that this ridicule, which affrights you, decreases very much when true love is opposed to it, and that through a mutual love we shall soon see it vanish. But, alas! where am I led by this arguments? This letter has a frightful length, and my heavy eyes bid me put an end to it. Good night then to the charming Isalina!

From the same to the same.
Oct. 22, 1779.

How sweet it is to steal an hour from sleep, and devote it to my friend! How precious these moments, if they effect a favourable turn to me. I proved yesterday, my dear Isalina, that ridicule is not so much to be feared as you seem to imagine, and that we shall find in ourselves sufficient means to repel it. Let us now see if we may so easily succeed in vanquishing the other obstacles which are like to prevent my happiness; the oppositions, I mean, of your parents and of my benefactress, besides our want of fortune.

As your parents are unknown to me, so are the views they may have for you settlement; but every thing bears the appearance of their having formed no project, and rather hoping, when delivered you up to the Countess Humieska, you would deserve so much of her Ladyship's concern, that she would provide you with an advantageous establishment. Thus our happiness depends only on our benefactress, and this idea affords me much comfort. Can we think she will oppose it? She looks on us as on her children, she bestows upon us maternal cares. We will fall at her feet, we will soften her, snatch her consent, and then all is done; we shall remain with her, we shall be indebted to her generosity for all we have; and through our earnest attentions and our gratitude we shall never cause her to repent the favours she has lavished upon us.

These, charming friend, are the reflections I have made for more than one year. I earnestly desire, that conscious of all their importance, you would draw the same consequences. I wish, above all, to convince you, that though your charms are deeply impressed on my heart, yet I did not yield to a blind passion, that I have attended to the probabilities and possibilities: thus you see that you have not quite bereft me of my wits, and there still remains enough to feel that I cannot be happy but on possessing my dear Isalina.

Isalina to Joujou.

October 24.

Indeed, my little friend, I know not how I shall answer you. I would not give you pain, yet I foresee that what I have to say must needs afflict you. You are very unreasonable, Joujou: yet I own, your arguments do much honour to your head and heart; but did I ever tell you I had a mind to marry? I can positively assure you I never had the least thought of it; and why should I? I am so happy, so gay, so tranquil: too young to find in the time past any subjects of affliction, and very little caring for the time to come, I enjoy the present in security. Be then afraid, let you should trouble my happiness; and if you have any friendship for me, give up those projects which cause me uneasiness. Nor would I have you grieve; be courageous and patient, you will soon acknowledge your madness, and thank me for having spoke to you as I do. Meanwhile be obliged to me for the kind sentiments which make me condescend to your whims, and answer letters I ought not to receive. Adieu Joujou; nevertheless I desire you to love me; remember I bid you do it; so obey, and prove to me that you are not a little ungrateful creature.

Isalina

Joujou to Isalina.

Nov. 1st, 1779.

O! my tender friend, all our projects overthrown, our happiness has disappeared. My benefactress disapproves of my sentiments. I know not how she has discovered them; but yesterday she spoke of them to me, and I thought it proper to seize that opportunity of confessing the whole, and asking of her favour which only can make me happy. At first she thought me joking; but in my extraordinary look, she soon saw I was but too much in earnest: my breath failed, my heart panted, my tears flowed abundantly. I thought I saw the moment in which her Ladyship, moved at my situation, would no longer oppose my felicity. I fell at her feet, I besought to yield to the motions of her beneficent heart. In vain she attempted to reason the case with me. I could not listen to her, I was in some measure out of my senses; upon which with a serious look she bade me go from her; but I could not leave her knees, and she was obliged to order a servant to take me away, and shut me up in my own apartment.

Here have I been these two days; I see nobody. The servant who waits on me drops not a single word; I understand he has been forbidden; but by the help of a few ducats, which luckily I had in my pocket, I have engaged him to tell me what was become of you. He answers me, that no one sees you; yet he has faithfully promised that this letter shall reach you. Ah! dear friend, if you feel any trouble, forgive me. I am the innocent cause of it. This misfortune may retard, but cannot annihilate our happiness; my love for you will gather new strength by it. Answer me, I pray. Consider that I shall not, I cannot receive any comfort but from you; that I would reject, and with indignation repel, such consolations as might be offered me from any one else. Only repeat that you approve of my sentiments, and, though I am confined and depressed, nobody can be happier than the enamoured

Joujou

Isalina to Joujou.

Nov. 4th.

Till now, Joujou, I held your passion, your projects, and our little intrigue only as a mere joke. I had suffered it through my being truly a friend to you, because I saw it made you happy, and, especially, because I was persuaded that it could have no fatal consequence. But, alas! I perceive that I am mistaken, and severely punished for it. How could I suspect that such a little being as you would be so obstinate, so enterprising? See to what I am exposed; everyone in the house talks of it; they banter you, and the counter-blow falls upon me. Besides, I bore the most severe reproaches from her Ladyship; it is in vain I tell her, that I am not an accomplice in your conduct, she makes me answerable for your madness, as if I had inspired you with it. Am I not punished enough for having sympathized with you? I always thought I loved you as a child; and who has ever seen that to love a child was deemed a crime? Endeavour then to retrieve all this, you may do it through your docility and submission; do not expose me any more to new troubles, and thereby convince me, that you sincerely desire the tranquillity and happiness of your

Isalina

Joujou to Isalina.

Nov. 5th, 1779

Your orders would have been sacred to me, dear Isalina, and, howsoever painful, I should have punctually executed them; but I am told, it is too late, and you have been cruelly sent back to your parents, whereby it is intended to separate us for ever. How could my benefactress determine on so violent an expedient? Yet by this, she only frustrates her own designs, and rivets me to you with indissoluble ties. On finding in me so steady a resolution, she will undoubtedly alter her sentiments, and we shall yet be happy. But will you pardon me the vexations I have caused you? Perhaps they will be a motive to hate me. No, charming friend, you cannot be so cruel; you would not pass an irrevocable verdict of unhappiness on the poor

Joujou

From the same to the same.

Nov. 10th, 1779.

I have, charming friend, just now appeared before my benefactress; she looked extremely meek and kind.

'Well! Joujou,' said she, 'have you made your reflections? I am sorry you have obliged me to use you so severely; but I am truly concerned for you, and I won't have you sacrifice your happiness to a foolish passion. I must interpose my authority to prevent it, if my counsels, if the gratitude you owe me cannot prevail on you.'

I could only answer with my tears, and she seemed mowed. 'Come, promise me,' rejoined she, 'to think no more of your love; on this condition I will forget all, and restore you to my friendship.'

'It does not lie in my power, Madame; judge of my love by my resistance; forgive me, I have consummated the unhappiness of Isalina, and nothing in the world can detach me from her.'

I saw that she was offended at my answer; I endeavoured to bring her back to herself, but it was too late. She ordered me to go out, and never to appear before her, until I had changed my sentiments. If on these terms only I am to see my benefactress again, I must grieve, indeed; but I shall see her no more. All pains are sufferable, except that of being separated from my dear Isalina. Meanwhile what does my love? Will she not let me hear from her? Has she entirely forgotten me? This is the only misfortune for which I should be inconsolable. Ah! charming friend, if you love me, if your constancy does not fail, we shall at last be happy. This is the most ardent wish of your tender and unfortunate

Joujou

Isalina to Joujou.
Nov. 11th.

I ought to hate you, Sir, after all that you make me endure. You are the cause that the Countess Humieska has withdrawn her bounty from me, and I have found myself under the afflicting necessity of repairing to my father's house. But that is not all. My mother loads me with reproaches; my sisters ridicule me. The whole town talk of this circumstance, and I cannot go anywhere, without being exposed to unpleasant and troublesome jokes. What then have I done Joujou, to cause me such violent vexations? You would force everybody to espouse your designs; but you will never accomplish it. Even were I inclined to live with you, my mother would by no means give her consent to an union she calls ridiculous and illmatched. She positively said so, and I assured her, that I never thought of it. Then give up, I entreat you, those pretensions; thereby appease Her Ladyship, to whom you are under so many obligations; silence the public talk, and restore me to the former gaiety you have robbed me of. On this condition only I shall remain your friend

Isalina

Joujou to Isalina.
Nov. 15, 1779

O! dear Isalina; what do you require of me? Must you be terrified at the least obstacle? Is our common happiness of so trifling a nature, as to give it up so easily? The public talk – and injuriously!.. Well! are you ignorant of the little importance of such talk? The public speak! It is not the world, it is only the despicable part of it, only the wicked, who upon the least appearances, pass rash judgments, and anticipate events, the wise wait for them, and are silent. But of what moment can such considerations be to us? If we constantly love one another, if you have the courage of uniting your fate to mine, shall we not have every body on our side? Ah! dear, friend, I fear nothing but your indifference and indecision. I am confined in my apartment as in a narrow prison, and have no other comfort, no other pleasure, than that of assuring my charming friend that I will always love her.

Joujou

Joujou to Isalina.
Nov. 20th.

At length, charming friend, my captivity is at the end. I have lost all for your sake, and should you not remain for me, I would.. yes, I would, indeed, give up my life.

This morning one of the chief officers of the Countess came from her Ladyship to tell me, that if I had not altered my resolution, I should go out of her house, never to return again. That is impossible, exclaimed I immediately; but on reflecting upon what conditions I could stay, I composed my mind, and coolly answered him I was ready to go out, and begged he would only tell my benefactress how much I was afflicted, to have incurred her displeasure. I besought her to pardon my resistance, and that I could never forget her bounty. Then I went out, and not without tears left a house wherein I had been so long as kindly used, as tenderly caressed as a dearly beloved child. How grievous such a predicament is to a heart susceptible of gratitude! I seem to be ungrateful.. I only am in love.

I knew not where to direct my steps, without money, without lodging, without resource. So dreadful was my situation! Love only supported my courage. It was he, undoubtedly, who inspired me with the thought of applying to Prince Casimir his Majesty's brother.[37] You know his affability, his mildness; you know, above all, the concern he always seemed to take in my affairs. My hopes have not been deceived: he knew all, except my departure, at which he was extremely surprised. 'Be not uneasy Joujou', said he to me 'you shall not be destitute, I will provide for you. Come and see me within a few days; I will speak of you with the king; you know he likes you, and I doubt not but he will grant you his protection'. These words reanimated my hopes. Yes, Isalina, if you will,

---

[37]   Kazimierz Poniatowski (1721–1800), Chamberlain of the Crown, elder brother of King Stanisław Augustus and his close political ally.

we may be happy; but can I not see you, speak to you, let you hear a thousand times, that until his last breath you shall be the only passion of the tender and faithful

Joujou

Joujou to Isalina.
November 25ᵗʰ

The Prince, my charming friend, sent for me this morning. How shall I express the gratitude with which he has impressed my heart? He asked me, whether I had a mind to enter into the Countess's house, and he would employ all her friends to prevail with her, or if I was still resolved to marry my dear Isalina? Such were his words. I answered him, that I excessively grieved for having lost the kindness of my benefactress, but the conditions upon which I might regain it were too hard for my heart. Then obtain the mother's consent, replied this beneficent Prince, and all the rest will go well. You see, my charming friend, you are thought to be the partner of my sentiments. I have been very cautious lest I should disclose that I have not yet obtained your consent; I had done amiss. Would you refuse it me, dear Isalina? Can you resolve to make him unhappy, who only aspires to promote your felicity? I shall be presented to the King, who has promised his illustrious brother to provide for me; thus no further inquietude for our subsistence. I am even permitted to hope for an annuity. Do then, my charming friend, bestow on me a ray of hope, and I will directly throw myself at your mother's feet. Will she not yield to my warm solicitations, especially on seeing me so illustriously protected? My supreme felicity depends on the sensibility of Isalina, and I expect it from her feeling heart; but let her remember, that the least indecision, the least delay, may cause all these glad hopes to vanish, and bring an everlasting unhappiness to her tender

Joujou

Isalina to Joujou.
November 26ᵗʰ

I was right when I said that this little tenacious Joujou would force everybody to comply with his own wishes: my mother too takes his part. She has read your two last letters, and is overjoyed to see you protected by the Prince Chamberlain:

her ambition is flattered by it, and she has declared to me, that I could not do better than to marry you. But, Joujou, do you understand it is she who says so, not I. Besides, she adds disagreeable reflections; she says, that our having caused so much talk, might prevent me from meeting with another establishment. But, dear mother, can I not be contented without a husband? Is there no living but in that state? Therefore you may see my mother when you please; she will give you her consent, as soon as you shall be assured of an annuity. But believe me, Joujou, all this cannot alter my resolutions; though you exert yourself to have a contract of marriage in due form, to have me sign it, to take me to church, and to marry me, you shall not cease, for all that, to be my little Joujou. Adieu, my friend; somewhere else you might be punished for thus forcing my inclination; here you must be loved, since one cannot hate you.

Isalina

Thus ends our correspondence. I waited upon Isalina's mother, whose consent I obtained. I saw my fair friend, whose inexhaustible stock of gaiety makes so happy a contrast with my temper, that I soon buried in oblivion all the vexations I had endured. The Prince Chamberlain kept his word; he was so kind as to present me to His Majesty, who approved of my marriage, and granted me an annuity of an hundred ducats.[38] The Pope's Nuncio wanted to prevent it, as being disproportionate; but the King prevailed over this obstacle, and some time after, the performance of the ceremony broke all the barriers that had been opposed to my felicity.

Yes, it is true, I have sacrificed for this happiness ease, riches, tranquillity. It has been for me the source of a thousand inquietudes, respecting either the subsistence of myself and family, or that of my children for the future. Yet, for these eight years that I have enjoyed it, I have found that nothing in the world is preferable to the satisfaction of pouring our inquietudes, our hopes, our fears into the bosom of a true friend united to our fate, whose tender and feeling soul relieves our pains by sharing them, and enlivens our pleasures with a far greater delight.

***

---

[38]   A ducat, otherwise known as a 'red złoty', was a coin minted in Poland, containing some 3.5 grams of gold.

I should have been too happy in my new state, if it had been possible that solely minding the present I had not cast an eye on the future; but man is not formed for pure and perfect felicity, disquietudes poison his enjoyments, and it but too often happens that from these very enjoyments arise his disquietudes. Notwithstanding my inexperience, I soon perceived that the King's favours would hardly be sufficient for our maintenance; and through much delicacy severely anticipating the necessities my new consort must submit to, the liveliness of my sentiments towards her still increased the bitterness and horror of my reflections. Although accustomed to the luxury and magnificence which had surrounded us in the palace of my benefactress, yet without grief, and even with a kind of pleasure, we should have embraced a middle station of life, the only one, perhaps, which gives to the tender and delicate sentiments their full scope and energy. But the question was not of expenses more or less considerable, we were likely to want even the necessaries of life; and I confess that the idea of seeing a beloved wife involved in misery, did not long permit me to enjoy the happiness of possessing her. To the great astonishment of all those who had deemed my marriage a folly, six weeks had scarce elapsed, when she apprised me of my being destined to be a father; and this news, which, if I had seen our subsistence secure, would have transported me with joy, did then only serve to sharpen of my uneasiness.

I was needful to take some step; but the choice was so much the more difficult, as having received no other education but such as was analogous to my size, and the station which the extreme bounty of Countess Humieska seemed to have ascribed to me, I possessed at most a few agreeable talents, which would not offer me any resource. In this perplexity my protectors were the first who suggested to me the idea of a second journey. The Prince Chamberlain, especially, seconded this project. He intimated to me, that having been kindly received in the principal Courts of Europe, when I was so happy as to accompany my benefactress, they would see me again with the same pleasure; and on knowing that I was a father, and without fortune, this position would increase the interest I had inspired, and in a decent manner procure me the means of leading, at my return, a peaceful and tranquil life.

Seduced by such a dazzling prospect, I entirely gave myself up to this idea. I spoke of it to the King, who not only vouchsafed to approve of my plan, but, even wishing to grant me a particular testimony of his bounty, ordered the Master of the Horse to supply me with a convenient coach. Having also taken all necessary measures, and being provided with letters of recommendation, I left Warsaw the 21ˢᵗ of November, 1780, and reached Cracow the 26ᵗʰ in the evening.

This town, formerly the capital of Poland, and where the coronation of the Kings was performed, is now no more than a frontier town, upon the Vistula, which separates what remains of Poland to the Commonwealth, from that part which the Austrians have invaded.[39] An illness having befallen my wife, we were obliged to stay there; and that indisposition having continued, the time came when she was brought to-bed, and delivered of a pretty little girl, whose birth made me experience feelings beyond description. Then I felt, on becoming a father, that though the passion which unites us to the object of our love, might before be ever so violent, yet it receives quite another energy from this new source of enjoyment.

As soon as my wife was recovered, I set out for Vienna, notwithstanding the cold which at that time was excessive. I only took care previously to have our coach set upon a sledge; and my wife, who could not part with the child, took, on her part, all necessary measures to keep it from the inclemency of the air, and to be able to suckle it without danger.

We reached Vienna on the 11ᵗʰ of February, 1781; but, unluckily for me, death had just before deprived the world of the illustrious Maria Theresa, that sovereign, whose noble and generous soul delighted in making happy all those who could get admittance to her. A mournful sorrow pervaded the whole town; and, as if every one had lost his wife, his parent, the deepest grief was impressed on all their features. All public entertainments, even concerts, were suspended. They only talked of the loss that had befallen them; of the magnanimity with which this heroine had supported adverse events. They recollected those disastrous times, when, forced to leave her residence, and holding her son in her arms, she had excited, amongst the Hungarians, that patriotic fermentation which had impelled them to do so much for her sake.[40] Whilst they expatiated

---

[39]   After the first partition (1772), in which the Polish-Lithuanian Republic lost close to one-third of its territory to Russia, Prussia, and Austria, the lands to the southeast of the Vistula River came under Austrian control.

[40]   This presumably refers to Maria Theresa's appearance before the Hungarian nobles at the diet, held in the royal castle at Pressburg/Pozsony (now Bratislava) in a dramatic moment

with complacency upon the means she had employed to re-establish her affairs, upon the glorious treaty which put an end to a war apparently threatening her in its origin with a total destruction;[41] on the other hand, with new regrets, enumerated the pains she had since taken, the cares she had been at to restore such of her provinces as had been desolated by war, to render the most advantageous to her subjects the peace she had procured them.

The general mourning did not prevent everybody from paying visits to each other; and I soon renewed my acquaintance with most of the nobleman I had the honour to see in my former travels. Even I may venture to say, that his Excellency the Prince de Kaunitz received my visit with every mark of benevolence and pleasure. He not only welcomed me kindly, but also permitted me to present my wife to him. He did us the honour to invite us to dinner, and would absolutely hasten his usual hour, which was between six and seven in the evening, not wishing, he said, to hurt his little friend's health. As that time his Imperial Majesty, Joseph II.[42] held no court, all the nobility assembled every evening in the Prince's hotel (where his relation, the C.[ountess] Clarissa,[43] received the guests). He did me so much favour as to present me to this assembly, and engage me often to come and spend the evening. There I had the honour to become acquainted with His Ex. Sir Robert Murray Keith,[44] the British Ambassador, who has been the principal cause afterwards of my passage into England. There also I had occasion to be convinced, that the great occupations of the Prince de Kaunitz, his superior talents, known to every one, in comprehending at one view

of the War of the Austrian Succession for the Habsburg monarchy and for the future empress herself, when her right to succeed her father Charles VI. The support of the Hungarians enabled her to regain Bohemia and Moravia from the Bavarian elector.

[41]   This probably refers to the peace treaty signed in Aachen after the War of the Austrian Succession in 1748. Although Austria lost Silesia it managed to safely emerge from a war that had threatened the existence of the entire Hapsburg monarchy. This was an undoubted success for Maria Theresa.

[42]   Joseph II (1741–1790), the son of Maria Theresa, Holy Roman Emperor (from 1765), co-regent (from 1765), and after his mother's death ruler of the countries of the Hapsburg monarchy.

[43]   It is hard to ascertain who Boruwłaski meant here. This is conceivably a reference to Marie Charlotte Questenberg, a close relative of Kaunitz's, but this is just conjecture given the difference in names.

[44]   Sir Robert Murray Keith (1730–1795), the British ambassador to Vienna (1772–1792), a skilled diplomat, polyglot, well known for his conversational talent.

the most extensive and complicate affairs, in foreseeing all their consequences, and preventing the events resulting from them, did not hinder him from looking on the minutest objects, the least worthy of fixing his attention. For having sent for the measure of my size, which he had carefully taken when I was in Vienna, in 1761,[45] with the Countess Humieska, he shewed to us, that from that time to 1781, I had grown upwards of ten inches. Which appeared as much surprising to those who, not having seen me before, did not conceive how this moment (1781) being hardly in size like a child four years old, I could have been ten inches shorter; as to those who, having seen me twenty years before, thought they observed in me as much difference, as there is between a youth of twelve and a grown man of thirty.[46]

Notwithstanding these fine appearances, and the professions of friendship I received everywhere, my journey did not answer the intended purpose; and the expenses occasioned by my stay at Vienna would have soon drained my resources, had not one of these uncommon friends, whose number unhappily is but small, in some manner forced me, on my setting out from Warsaw, to accept of a letter of credit, which I made use of. My hopes, it is true, were grounded upon a concert; but though I must have waited 'till the mourning was over, yet I had still new difficulties to overcome, new obstacles to surmount. A crowd of *Virtuosi* were inscribed on the catalogue, at the royal theatre; and if I had been obliged to wait for my turn, I might have been kept a great way back. Happily for me, my protectors in general, and especially Mr. Gunter, Secretary to his Imperial Majesty, so much pressed Mr. Dorval, the manager of the house, that I was preferred before the others; and they were even so kind as to manage for me, and conduct the concert and the expenses.

I was so fortunate as to be honoured with a numerous assembly, and almost all the nobility was present. I attempted in a short speech to express my gratitude to them. I wanted likewise to make an apology before that same nobility, who, twenty years ago, having seen me surrounded with the eclat of greatness, saw me now reduced to the sad necessity of appearing in public. Love, an adored wife, a child, the precious fruit of our union, pleaded in my favour; they seemed satisfied

---

[45] Boruwłaski's dating is off here: other sources indicate that he was in Austria with Humiecka in 1759 at the latest.

[46] Whereas in reality this was the difference in his height between 20 years old and more than 40.

with my compliment, and I experienced all the indulgence of the public, who undoubtedly bestowed their applause, rather on my earnest desire of pleasing them, than on my talents.

I was at that time very far from thinking, that, through necessity of providing for the most essential wants of life, I should be obliged to expose myself to view for money. The education I had received, the manner in which I had lived 'till now, contributed to make me look upon this resource as beneath me; and though all the persons concerned for my welfare endeavoured to bring me to that resolution, yet I had still much reluctance to take it. Above all, the Baron de Breteuil, then ambassador from the court of France to that at Vienna,[47] was incessantly pressing me thereon. This nobleman, equally known for his penetration, and the brilliant career he has run, said to me one day: 'Do not think, my little friend, that concerts will always be sufficient to answer your expenses, and to procure you a support; you must needs give up pride, or choose misery; and if you do not intend to lead the most unhappy life; if you wish to enjoy, in future, a state of tranquillity, it is indispensable you should resolve to make exhibition of yourself.' The next day the Prince de Kaunitz spoke to me in the same manner amidst a crowded levee. His Excellency, Sir Robert Murray Keith was present, he prevailed upon me to go over to England, in preference to France, which was country I intended first to visit. The Prince supported this advice, and earnestly desired the Ambassador to interest himself for me. His Excellency promised me letters of recommendation to the greatest personages at the British Court; the Prince made him an acknowledgement for it, and assured him he would seek every opportunity to shew him how sensible he was of all was done to his little friend.

If all these reasons did not entirely prevail, at least they acted upon me; and I resolved to leave Vienna, being supplied with the best letters of recommendation to many Princes of Germany. But before I speak of the kind welcome I met with the several Courts I visited, I think it a duty to mention the beneficence of the Countess Féguetté,[48] who insisted on my not setting out till I had previously

---

[47]   Louis Auguste le Tonnelier baron de Breteuil (1730–1807), French diplomat and ambassador to Vienna.

[48]   This probably means the Countess Fekètè, the wife of the Hungarian aristocrat Janos Fekètè.

made a journey to Presbourg[49] the capital of Hungary; and not only defrayed all the expenses of this tour, but even added a present of thirty ducats. I staid there only the necessary time to give a concert; and from thence I went to Lintz, where the Count de Thierheim,[50] Governor of Low Austria, and son-in-law to the Prince de Kaunitz, loaded me with kindness. He was so good as to lend me for the concert his band of musicians: this band was composed of fifteen young men, all good performers, the eldest of whom was not seventeen. The audience being very thinly attended, occasioned this to be said: 'Little concert, little music, little players, and little receipt.'

I ought not to omit a charming and ingenious saying of the Countess de Thierheim, then between six and seven.[51] This fine young lady did not cease to look at me all the concert; when it was over, she ran to her papa, and clinging round his neck, earnestly begged he would buy her this little man.

'Well! what would you do with him, my dear child?' said the Count to her, 'besides we have no apartment for him.'

'Let that be no obstacle, papa,' replied she, 'I will keep him in mine, will take the utmost care of him, have the pleasure of dressing and adoring him, of loading him with caresses and dainties.' In a word, they had much ado to persuade her that it was not possible to purchase the little man like a doll.

The next place where I stopped at was Ratisbon;[52] but not finding the Prince de la Tour and Taxis,[53] who was then at his estate at Teschen,[54] I went immediately to Munich, where Her Royal Highness the Electress Dowager,[55] whom I had the honour to visit twenty years before, was very glad to see me

---

[49]   Under the Hapsburgs, Pressburg (now Bratislava, the capital of Slovakia) served as the capital of Hungary and was the seat of the governing council, the central instrument of power, and representatives of the Hungarian estates also gathered there.

[50]   Christoph Wilhelm Thürheim (1731–1809), husband of the Kaunitz's daughter Marie Antoinette, then no longer alive in 1781.

[51]   Given that Marie Antoinette Thürheim had died in 1769, her daughter must have been somewhat older than Boruwłaski claims and been around 12 years old.

[52]   Regensburg in Bavaria, from 1661 the permanent seat of the Reichstag of the Holy Roman Empire.

[53]   Karl Anselm, Prince of Thurn and Taxis (1733–1805).

[54]   A city on the Olza River that belonged to the Hapsburg monarchy, now divided between Poland (Cieszyn) and the Czech Republic (Těšín).

[55]   Maria Anna (1728–1797), the daughter of Augustus III King of Poland, the widow of Bavarian Elector Maximilian Joseph.

again, and shewed me the same kindness as at the time of my former journey. She perfectly remembered the particular pleasure her illustrious husband had in conversing with me, and the special favour he had done me with the gift of a beautiful ivory case turned by himself, and to which were set golden circles enriched with small diamonds. She presented me to His Most Serene Highness, the now reigning Elector.[56] I was often invited to the assemblies at Court, and every time I was the subject of general conversation. They took great pleasure in tracing back many events and circumstances of my former appearance in that town; this in particular, when at the assembly, several charming ladies were eager to take me on their lap and clasp me in their arms: I could not help observing to them that, being twenty-two, and a child only in size, their fond caresses made me endure the most cruel torment. His Most Serene Highness was so good as to appoint a day for the concert, all the expenses of which he desired to clear, and made me, besides, a present in money. Her Royal Highness, the Electress Dowager, also made a present of a handsome gold box filled with ducats.

After having taken my leave of their Highnesses, I directed my route to Teschen, where being arrived, I sent to the Prince de la Tour and Taxis, that I might be permitted to pay my respects to him. He answered, that he had often seen men of my species, and had no curiosity to see any more, except one who had travelled with the Countess Humieska, whom he had always desired to see, without ever having had it in his power. When he was told that I was not only the very same he had desired to meet with, but even that I was the bearer of letters from the Princess his daughter,[57] and the Prince Radziwiłł his son in law,[58] which would confirm the fact, he ordered a coach and fix, with an equerry, to bring me to his palace.

After having bowed to the Prince and all his court, I approached His Highness, and told him that one of the most charming ladies in the world had charged me to embrace him with all my heart. Without giving me time to finish my phrase, the Prince lifted me up in his arms, saying: "T is with great pleasure,

---

56　Karl Teodor Wittelsbach (1724–1799), Bavarian Elector (from 1777) after his predecessor's heirless death.

57　Princess Sophie of Thurn and Taxis (1758–1800), the daughter of Karol Anselm and the wife of Hieronim Wincenty Radziwiłł.

58　Hieronim Wincenty Radziwiłł (1759–1786), the son of Michał Kazimierz, Chamberlain of Lithuania.

my little man.' Then having put me on the ground again, he asked me, who had
charged me with so agreeable a commission? I immediately delivered to him
the letters of the Prince his son-in-law, and of the Princess his daughter; and
told him that, the day before my setting out from Warsaw, having waited on
the Princess to receive her orders, she had been so kind as to embrace me, and
say, it was on condition I would return this kiss to her papa. She afterwards had
enjoined me to press him to take a trip to Poland, to see a daughter who loved
him tenderly, and to whose happiness his presence only was wanting. Should
he not determine on it, nothing could hold her back; but she would set out
immediately, not being able to live any longer without the pleasure of seeing
him. During all this recital, the Prince's sensibility was not equivocal, his eyes
sparkled with tears, and, after having read the letters, he embraced me again,
asked many questions of the manner I had parted from the Countess Humieska,
of my marriage, of what had induced me to undertake new travels; and, seeming
satisfied with my answers, he said: 'You must needs be fatigued, go to rest, I will
give orders that you want nothing; it will be proper for you to spend here four
or five days, to walk about and enjoy the benefit of the air.' When I went home I
saw that the Prince's orders had preceded me. They brought me from him wines
of every kind, and during four or five days I staid at Teschen, there was nothing
but feasts and entertainments. In fine, when I took my leave of His Highness,
he engaged me to pay a visit to the Prince de Wallerstein[59] his son-in-law, who
at that time resided at Honnaltheim,[60] his county seat. This proposal being too
agreeable to be refused, I accepted; and the Prince not only added to so many
favours a present in gold, but I also found, at my return to my inn, that all my
expenses had been paid, and the Prince had ordered post-horses to conduct me
to Dillingen,[61] where I had left my baggage.

   Being arrived at Honnaltheim, I was presented to the Prince de Wallerstein,
by whom, considering the recommendation I had from his father-in-law, I could
not fail to be kindly received. But though he welcomed me with all the affability
and politeness imaginable, I soon perceived that he was labouring under a dark
melancholy, and seemed to value life only for his extreme attachment to this

---

[59]   Kraft Ernst, Prince of Oetingen-Wallerstein (1748–1802).
[60]   Hohenaltheim, the town in Bavaria that served as the summer residence of the
Princes of Oettingen-Wallerstein.
[61]   Dillingen an der Donau, a Bavarian town.

Princess his daughter, then four years old.[62] I was soon informed of the cause of this sadness, in which all his court took the greatest concern; and my astonishment ceased when I was told, that the moment which made him a father, deprived him of a charming and adored consort,[63] for whom he had mourned ever since. She who was to complete his happiness, had plunged him into this state of apathy and insensibility, subsequent to the most violent ravings, which had alarmed his court, first for his life, and afterwards for his senses. Yet, notwithstanding this sadness, as my figure and manners seemed to amuse the young Princess, and nothing could make any impression upon him but what interested this child. The Prince did me the honour to attend my concert; and when I took leave, he was pleased to present me with a very pretty enamelled watch.

Till then I had no reason but to applaud myself for the expedient I had taken of travelling; I had everywhere been seen with pleasure, and met with much civility. But nothing can be compared to the reception I found at the Court of His Most Serene Highness the Margrave of Anspach,[64] at Triersdorff;[65] nor can I find expressions strong enough to describe the sentiments of respectful gratitude I shall always have for this amiable Prince, whose generous treatment has made the deepest impressions on my heart. 'T is to the Mademoiselle Clairon I am indebted for it; and with the greatest pleasure do I embrace this opportunity of paying her my homage for such a favour. That distinguished actress, after having acquired so universal and so well merited a reputation, seeking only to enjoy a peaceful and easy life in the circle of a chosen society, spent every summer at Triersdorff, where she was detained by the kindness, I may say the tender friendship His Highness honoured her with.[66] Having had the advantage of being acquainted with her at Paris in my first travels, she saw me again with new pleasure, and was so obliging as to present me to the Margrave. She represented

---

62   Friedericke Sophie Therese, Princess of Oettingen-Wallerstein (1776–1831).

63   Maria Theresia, Princess of Thurn and Taxis (1757–1776), daughter of Karol Anselm, married the Prince of Wallerstein in 1774 and died in childbirth after two years of marriage.

64   Charles Alexander, Margrave of Brandenburg-Ansbach-Bayeruth (1736–1806).

65   Triesdorf, the summer residence of the margraves of Ansbach.

66   This friendship was undoubtedly very tender indeed: the margrave had met and fallen in love with Mademoiselle Clarion when he was visiting Paris incognito in 1770. He persuaded her to come to Ansbach, where she lived as his mistress for a total of 17 years (1770–1787).

to him, in so affecting and lively a manner, the difference of my present situation from what I had enjoyed when protected by the Countess Humieska, that she inspired this good Prince with that uncommon interest he has since taken in me. I had the honour to partake of his table almost every day; after dinner I was admitted to play at shittle-cock[67] with Her Highness;[68] and, as I was tolerably skilful in this exercise, which suits my size so well, they seemed to take great pleasure in seeing me play. The Princess would also give my wife some particular marks of kindness; she presented her with a handsome and complete dress, and gave me a snuff-box, together with a small ring of the most exquisite taste. In fine, I passed six weeks in that delightful place, amidst pleasures, entertainments, and that friendly protection which is so flattering when it comes from the great. I cannot remember without feeling the utmost sense of endless gratitude, with what good nature Their Highnesses offered to take care of my daughter. I do not cease to praise the blessed day that procured me so illustrious a benefactor, when I recollect how earnest this good Prince was to calm my inquietudes for the fate of this child; and that on perceiving her mother's grief to part with an only child, he deigned to address me with these remarkable words, which are still echoed to the bottom of my heart: 'My friend, it is not only a Prince's word I give you to take care of your child, receive that of an honest man, and be assured that I will provide for her.'

O! my daughter, I shall leave you no inheritance. Reduced incessantly to struggle with fortune, your father is compelled to seek for every possible means of providing for his subsistence; but here he bequeaths you to the sacred word of a magnanimous Prince, and, should you know how to value so great a favour, your happiness must necessarily be the consequence.

Some days after we prepared to set out, and on taking our leave, Her Highness deigned to give us repeated assurances of the fate of our child. The Prince, to complete all his favours, presented me with a purse of forty luis-d'ors,[69] under the pretence of paying the expenses of my journey. I could not make any other return but my tears, for so many tokens of beneficence, and it was with the bitterest

---

67 Shuttle-cock, a popular game of the time, similar to badminton.
68 Caroline Friederike von Sachsen-Coburg-Saalfeld, Margravine of Ansbach (1735–1791)
69 A French coin containing approx. 6.8–7.3 grams of gold.

regret I tore myself from a place which I had so much reason to be partial to, which everything has contributed to render interesting to me.

On leaving Triersdorff, my only care was to hasten my journey, that I might reach England as soon as possible, I have already observed that His Excellency Sir Robert Murray Keith had prevailed upon me to take this route, by having assured me a thousand times that I could not fail of making a brilliant fortune, in a country where generosity and greatness of soul are reckoned among the characteristic virtues of the nation.

Therefore, after having passed rapidly through Francfort, Mayence,[70] and Manheim, I went to Strasbourg, where I had the honour to give a concert to Her Highness the Princess Christina,[71] for whom I had a letter from her sister, the Electress of Bavaria. She was so kind as to engage me often to spend the evening at her court, and the day before my departure, she presented me with a handsome gold box of three different colours, which she ordered to be made on purpose for me, and which necessity has obliged me to part with since I came to London.

Afterwards I directed my course to Brussels, where I had the honour to be presented to Their Royal Highnesses the Governor and Governess of the Low Countries.[72] All the nobility there welcomed me with much kindness, and I was even permitted to give my concert in the elegant room, which they have caused to be erected for their assemblies, and wherein all the expenses are their charge. I staid at Brussels only a few days, thence I came to Ostend, where I intended to embark.

I had never been at sea, nor even beheld that proud element; therefore one may imagine the emotions of surprise, admiration and fear, with which I was agitated at the sight of such an awful spectacle, such a depth and extent of boisterous waters, upon which I was soon to expose my own life, and what I held dearest in the world. I considered the main as likely to be my grave; and my

---

[70]   Mainz, the largest city of Rhineland-Palatinate.

[71]   Maria Christina of Saxony (1735–1782), daughter of the Saxon Elector, Polish King Augustus III.

[72]   In 1782, when Boruwłaski visited, Belgium (then known as the Austrian Netherlands) was under the rule of the emperor, on whose behalf power was exercised by governors-general; in 1782 this was Albrecht Casimir, Prince of Sachsen-Teschen (1738–1822).

apprehensions were very nearly realized. During a passage of four days we were continually tossed in storms, our masts broke, our sails were carried away; and if to my own situation is added that which I suffered for the state of my wife, who was afflicted with great sickness and spitting of blood which nothing could stop. One may conceive the satisfaction I felt on our getting out of the packet. We landed at Margate, the 20th of March 1782, and a few days after set out for London, where we arrived without any other accident.

We had brought with us a number of recommendatory letters to many of the first nobility. I immediately made use of those directed to their Graces Duke and Duchess of Devonshire[73]; and though I had everywhere heart them praised for their politeness, their affability, their desire of obliging, yet I soon learnt by myself that true merit is always superior to the highest renown. This illustrious couple received me most graciously, and condescended to say, that having been informed of some of my misfortunes, they desired I would have recourse to them if I wanted any thing. The Duchess afterwards asked me many questions, with that affability and feeling concern, which, far from denoting an eager curiosity, only wait for answers that may give occasion to bestow favours. In effect, having been informed that I was not lodged conveniently, and that for want of speaking the language, I could hardly provide for my necessaries, she immediately gave orders to procure me a comfortable lodging at her own expense; this we held some month. The very next day Her Grace having been informed that my wife was ill, sent Dr. Walker to attend her; and I esteem this not to be smallest favour of the Duchess, to have procured me the acquaintance of so respectable a gentleman, whose friendship to me has not ceased, since my arrival in England, bestowing upon me and my family, his cares and remedies with generosity, in a manner that puts it entirely out of my power to acknowledge as I would, and leaves me only this opportunity of publicly professing how far my gratitude extends.

The first visit of Dr. Walker was pleasant enough. The Duchess had not informed him of the species of man whose wife she desired him to attend; and on coming into the apartment he took me for a child. Being near his patient's bed, he was taken up with asking her questions, and I, on my part, with thanking him, recommending the care of my wife; and as the tone of my voice is much above my stature, so he was at a loss to conceive from whence came the speech

---

73   William Cavendish, Duke of Devonshire (1748–1811), and his wife Georgiana.

that was directed to him. My wife perceiving his embarrassment, told him who I was; but he could hardly be persuaded, either that I am a man, or that the voice he had heard could come from such a diminutive being.

Some days after I was astonished at the entrance of a taylor, who saying he was sent by the Duke of Devonshire, presented me with some charming habiliments, containing a complete suit, the principal of which was, a superb coat embroidered with gems and silver, and the rest in proportion, besides a very handsome steel sword. On waiting upon His Grace to return him my thanks, I had the honour to be presented to Lady Spencer,[74] who very kindly appointed a day where I might pay her my respects at Her Ladyship's house. I met there with His Royal Highness the Prince of Wales,[75] to whom Her Ladyship was so good as to present me, and he spoke to me with that affability which gains him every heart. When I retired, Her Ladyship made me accept a *rouleau* of thirty guineas,[76] and the next day His Royal Highness sent me a very pretty little watch.

A short time after my arrival in London there came also a stupendous giant. He was eight feet three or four inches high, English measure.[77] His shape was very well proportioned, his physiognomy agreeable; and, what is very uncommon in men of this sort, his strength was equal to his size. He was at that time only two and twenty. Many persons seemed desirous of seeing us together; my protectors, the Duke and Duchess of Devonshire, being one day to see him, in company with Lady Spencer, they were so kind as to take me with them. Our surprise was, I think, equal. The giant remained a moment speechless, viewing me with looks

---

[74] There were two ladies of this name whom Boruwłaski might have met visiting the Duchess of Devonshire – her mother Georgiana Spencer (–1814), the wife of John, the first Count of Spencer, or her sister-in-law Lavinia (–1831), from March 1781 the wife of Georgiana's brother John, the second Count of Spencer. This reference is most likely to the elder Lady Spencer, who maintained close ties to her daughter.

[75] The heir to the throne, the future George IV, King of Great Britain from 1820.

[76] The English monetary system was quite complex at that time: one gold guinea contained about 8.5 grams of gold and was equivalent to 21 shillings, a pound was equal to 20 shillings (or about 8 grams of gold), and a crown was equivalent to 5 shillings. A shilling was a silver coin and was divided into 12 pence.

[77] The publisher of the 1902 edition of Boruwłaski's memoirs identifies this as Patrick O'Brien (*c.*1760–1804), but O'Brien was in London in 1784, whereas Boruwłaski seems to have met a different 'Irish giant': Charles Byrne (1760–1783), who is known to have been in London at the time stated in the memoirs (late 1782/early 1783), was 2.49 metres tall, and like Boruwłaski showed himself publicly for money.

of astonishment; then stooping very low to present me his hand, which would easily have contained a dozen like mine, he made me a very polite compliment. Had a painter been present, the contrast of our figures might have suggested to him the idea of an interesting picture; for having come near him, the better to show the difference, it appeared that his knee was nearly upon a level with the top of my head.

About this time I was visited by a gentleman, from whose appearance, agreeable conversation, affable and easy countenance, though he did not make himself known, it was easily perceived that nobility was his. I soon found him to be His Royal Highness the Duke of Gloucester,[78] at whose door I had called, as soon as I arrived, to deliver a letter which His Highness the Margrave of Anspach had favoured me with for His Royal Highness. But as I had not been fortunate enough to meet him, he was unknown to me; and it was Mr. Cramer,[79] the first violin engaged in His Majesty's concert, who having come to see me, met with His Royal Highness, and thus preventing his remaining any longer incognito, gave him an opportunity of speaking to me of the letter I had left for him, assuring me that such a recommendation should have very great influence with him, and I might depend he would do all in his power to oblige me. From that time this amiable Prince has not ceased to favour me with unequivocal proofs of his generosity and protection. Unhappy for me, I was not long to enjoy his bounties; the epoch of His Royal Highness' travels was fixed, and I felt the mortification of seeing him set out soon after my arrival. But I should be deficient in the duty incumbent upon me through respect and gratitude, were I not to publish his having deigned to give me a call even on the day before his departure, to supply me with new testimonies of his beneficence; he left me only to regret my having known so powerful and so generous a Protector so short a time.

The Duchess of Devonshire, on her side, as well as her whole family, still continued to take the most lively interest in all that related to me. Well knowing that my situation was beneath my birth, education and sentiments, and consulting

---

[78]   William Henry, Duke of Gloucester (1743–1805), the grandson of George II, the third son of Frederick Louis, Prince of Wales, the younger and favourite brother of George III.

[79]   Wilhelm Cramer (*c.*1745–1799), a violinist from a family of musicians from Mannheim. A member of the Royal Society of Musicians from 1777.

only the feelings of her heart, she recommended me to all her acquaintance; and if I am not perfectly happy, it is not that Her Grace has neglected to do every thing in her power. But what I can never forget, and for which I must always entertain for her the most dutiful respect, the most grateful sense, is that I was, through her kind interposition, introduced to most of the nobility, amongst whom I have met with protectors, even I may say, with friends, who have had for me so great a regard, that I cannot find words to express with the remembrance of their favours.

Yet I should be wanting in my duty towards Mr. de Bukaty[80] the Minister of His Majesty the King of Poland, if I neglected to declare here, that I am indebted to him for my being known to His Excellency the Count Bruhl,[81] and to Lady Countess of Egremont,[82] who since has never ceased to show me the truest concern. It is to her I am beholden for having been presented to Their Majesties. Her Ladyship having been informed that I was spoken of at Court, had the goodness to send for one of my shoes, got it stuffed with cotton, that she might show it to the Queen; and this having excited curiosity, Their Majesties were graciously pleased to appoint a day for the purpose of seeing me.

It was on the 23d of May, 1782, that my respectable Protectress was so kind as to take me to Her Majesty.[83] The King[84] and all the Royal Family were present. His Majesty condescended to bid me sit down, and asked me many questions, both about my travels, and the manner how I became acquainted with his Ambassador at Vienna.[85] H.R.H. the Prince of Wales often interrupted the conversation by witty and agreeable sallies; and the young Princes and Princesses recovered from their first astonishment I had caused them, entered with me into that familiarity which characterises youth. In fine, I had the honour to stay four hours with Their Majesties; and, having used all my efforts to please them, I

---

80   Franciszek Bukaty (1747–1797), the Polish *chargé d'affaires* in London (from 1772), later minister plenipotentiary (1789–1793).

81   Count Hans Moritz Brühl (1736–1809), the Saxon ambassador in London (from 1764).

82   Alice Marie Carpenter (–1794), the wife first of Count Charles Wyndham Egremont, then after his death of Moritz Brühl (from 1767).

83   Sophia Charlotte of Mecklenburg-Strelitz (1744–1818), wife of George III and Queen of Great Britain (from 1761).

84   George III (1738–1820), King of Great Britain from 1760.

85   Sir Robert Murray Keith.

enjoyed the satisfaction of seeing that, in some respect, I had not failed in my aim.

These exertions, however, were near being fatal to me; I came home with fever, and the very next day fell dangerously ill. His Majesty did me the favour to send his physician Sir Richard Jebb,[86] by whose care, together with those of our good friend Dr. Walker, I recovered in a fortnight.

The public have spoken very freely with regard to that visit; it has even been mentioned in some newspapers, that I received from Their Majesties a considerable sum of money; but it is with this report as with many others which are founded on conjectures only. If it had had the least foundation in truth, I would not have omitted any of its particulars; as I consider it my duty to declare all the favours I have been indulged with. The fact is, that His Majesty vouchsafed to treat me as a Polish gentleman; and though there be no humiliation in receiving presents from a great Lord, though it is an honour to receive some from a King; yet I have been more flattered with this mark of distinction His Majesty was pleased to show me, than if he had made me come to his palace merely as an object of curiosity.

However, every proud sentiment must be silent, when the matter in question is to provide for the subsistence of those who are dearest to us; and it was soon necessary that this last consideration should prevail with me above all others. Besides, though it were possible to have always recourse to generous benefactors, do we not experience more painful, more humiliating sentiments, in incessantly importuning them, than if by some other means we could succeed in procuring ourselves a decent maintenance?

Such were the reflections which arose in my mind from my own situation, and which met with the approbation of those to whom I communicated them. They advised me to give concerts; afterwards they prevailed upon me to make an exhibition from myself, first at one guinea, then a five shillings, then at half a crown, when the pressure of want, and call of nature had stifled in my heart all that seemed shocking to me in such an expedient.

But let us not anticipate events; I beg the indulgence of my readers, and wish to demonstrate that my conduct has always been the effect of necessity, and

---

[86] Richard Jebb (1729–1789), baronet (from 1778), physician to the Prince of Wales (from 1780), from 1786 physician to the king.

that I have in a particular manner experienced the generosity of my protectors. Though it has not proved sufficient to save any sum out of it to secure me a competency, nevertheless this generosity has been carried very far, since through it I have been decently supported during six years that I have lived in England, where, being obliged to keep apartments at a high rent, to make many excursions, and often to repeat them, and to lay out large sums of money for my concerts, I could not help, in spite of my private oeconomy, spending between four and five hundred [pounds] a year.

The first concert I gave was at Carlisle House, Soho. My respectable Protectress, always anxious for my welfare, was frightened at the expense it occasioned me, and which actually amounted to eighty guineas; but I was amply indemnified, the assembly being both brilliant and numerous; and if that enthusiasm had continued, some concerts given now and then would have been sufficient to set me above mediocrity: this however did not happen; for having attempted a few weeks after to give another at the same place, I scarcely cleared my expenses. Half the nobility were gone to the country, the others were departing, and I was obliged to think of new means of support.

At the beginning of the Winter following I went to Bath, where I met with most of my protectors, and had the honour of becoming acquainted with a very amiable family, Mr. and Mrs. Harbouin, who had a great regard for me, and shewed me much kindness, for which I shall always entertain the most grateful sense. I gave at Bath a breakfast, which was very brilliant and agreeable, Mr. Harbouin was so obliging as to cause two hundred tickets to be distributed among his friends and acquaintance, and it was with the utmost pleasure he brought me this small sum a few days after the breakfast.

At my return to London, respect and gratitude led me to the door of the Duchess of Devonshire, and I cannot say to what degree I was affected, on perceiving, that notwithstanding many attempts, it was impossible for me to obtain admittance. I was afraid I had incurred Her Grace's displeasure; and the vexation occasioned by such an idea began to impair my health, when Lady Clermont[87] restored my mind to tranquillity, by assuring me that this powerful protectress still entertained the same sentiments for me, and I should soon be convinced of it.

---

[87]   Frances Fortescue, Countess of Clermont (*c.*1734–1820).

This conversation recalled to my mind what several Lords, who about six months before met at my apartment, made me hope for. The design was to open subscription, at the head of which the most illustrious of my Protectors would be put, to secure me an easy and decent maintenance for the remainder of my days. They had come so often to question me upon this subject, and the concern they seemed to have for me was so evident, that for a while I ventured to flatter myself that this project would take place; and, indeed, I should have esteemed myself very happy, if by that means I had been indebted to the first English nobility for my welfare. But I was destined to be the sport of fate; and whether other affairs hindered those who at first wished to undertake this business for me, or that they thought it was not yet time, the subscription did not take place.

Some time after I heard of the happy delivery of the Duchess of Devonshire.[88] I was overjoyed at this event, and no longer questioned the motive of my having been refused admittance to Her Grace's apartment.

It was about this time, as the visits, which were still at five shillings, were insufficient to defray my expenses, so I determined to give a concert, which was performed in one of Mr. Gallini's assembly-rooms, in Hanover-square.[89] Many of my protectors were so kind as to take upon them to distribute my tickets; and His Royal Highness the Prince of Wales deigned to assure me positively he would assist at it; but unluckily, other engagements prevented him from doing me that honour. Lord Townshend[90] wished to do everything for me in this circumstance; but through the circumspection inseparable from the place he then occupied, he could not put himself forward, confined himself to attend my concert, with all his family, and sent me twenty-five guineas for five tickets he had taken.

---

[88] On 12 July 1783 the first child of the Duke and Duchess of Devonshire was born – to the Duke's disappointment it was not a son but a daughter, Georgiana Dorothy Cavendish (–1858).

[89] Giovanni Andrea Battista Gallini (1728–1805), a teacher of dancing from Florence, very popular in London. He built a concert hall on Hanover Square (the Concert Rooms), which he rented out for various events. He figured in a romantic love story with the elder daughter of the Earl of Abington, who fell for him and left her family home to marry him.

[90] This probably means Lord Thomas Townshend (1733–1800), Viscount of Sydney (from 1783), who at the time described by Boruwłaski was home secretary, the cabinet's chief spokesman in parliament, and *de facto* the leader of the House of Commons.

This concert having made me a little more easy in my circumstances, I left London and set out for Ireland, in the month April 1783.[91] This trip was longer than I at first imagined, as I staid two months at Bristol and Chester, where the attentions and marks of friendship bestowed on me by all Mrs. Blackburne's family, detained me seven weeks.

It was during my stay there, I got acquainted with one of those men, who, having received of nature wit and good appearance, think themselves exempt from being principled with honour and uprightness, and who, compelled through their want of conduct to leave their own country, establish their resources in foreign lands, upon the credulity and good faith of those whom they find means to inspire with confidence. This man assumed the name of Marquis de Montpellier, and for a while was very cautious not to come to my apartments but among great folks, with whom he strove to act an officious part, in order to give me a good opinion of his connections. Nor did he fail in his design; as he had artfully persuaded me that he entertained intimacy with the first nobility of Ireland; that, if he would attempt it, nothing could be so easy for him as to procure me there a subscription of two thousand five hundred guineas; that for this purpose he had only to set out before me, to secure a house, and announce my coming, in order to prepare their minds for my reception. So I could not help giving credit to all the chimeras he lulled me with, in spite of the observations of a true friend,[92] in whom I should have trusted more, considering his experience, and the good counsels he had not ceased to give me since my departure from Warsaw. Thus the Marquis set out, having my full powers; and I followed him a fortnight after. We had a fortunate passage; and as Lady Clermont had condescended to give me a letter for the master of the packet, I had much reason to be pleased with the attentions and cares of the captain and all his crew, who notwithstanding my entreaties, however pressing I was, would not accept even the least gratification for their trouble. On my arrival at Dublin I hoped

---

[91]   Boruwłaski's dating is off here: he cannot have left for Ireland in April, since his own daughter was born in London in May, as reported in the press, and it was also in London that he received the news of the birth of the Duchess of Devonshire's daughter in July. He most likely departed in mid-August – an announcement of his arrival to Bristol has survived, dated 25 August.

[92]   According to the publisher of the 1902 edition of the memoirs, H.R. Heatley, this refers to Isalina's uncle, Mr de Trouville.

to have found a house ready for me; but was extremely surprised at meeting my fellow in an inn near the port, where he had announced me for a great Lord, and, thanks to his provident cares, I fared very daintily, not yet perceiving that I was his dupe. Nay, it was not till a fortnight after, that being informed by respectable persons, both of the pretended Marquis's character, and the harm that such an acquaintance would do me, I had resolution enough to get rid of this parasite, by giving him money to cross the sea again.

When I set out from London, my protectors had been so attentive as to supply me with letters of recommendation, as well to His Grace the Lord Lieutenant,[93] as to the chief Lords and most of the distinguished Ladies in Ireland; through which means, during two years I staid there, I should have met with every kind of pleasures, had not all my enjoyments been frustrated by my wife's impaired state of health, whom I had been obliged to leave in England, and who, having four months afterwards come to meet me, was still in a languishing condition. My Lord Vice-Roy sent for me to his Court on an assembly day, and was graciously pleased to make me a present of twenty guineas. Some time after he was succeeded by His Grace the Duke of Rutland,[94] under whose patronage and that of the Duchess,[95] I had the honour to give the Irish nobility a concert and a ball at the Rotunda,[96] in May 1784. The assembly was extremely brilliant; Her Grace the Vice-Reine was its principal ornament, not only for her rank and beauty, but still more through that elegance and affability with which she knows so well how to grace all her actions. She was graciously pleased to open the Ball, which she did with a gaiety that attracted the applause of all the assembly; and

---

[93]   Lord Lieutenant of Ireland, the representative of the king (or 'viceroy'). At this time (from May 1783 to February 1784) this was Robert Henley, Earl of Northington (1747–1786).

[94]   Charles Manners, Duke of Rutland (1754–1787), a politician, friend of William Pitt, and Lord Lieutenant of Ireland from 11 February 1784.

[95]   Mary Isabella Somerset (1756–1831), the youngest daughter of Charles, Duke of Beaufort, from 1775 the wife of Charles Manners, was indeed considered a very beautiful woman, and in this and other regards was the most serious rival to the Duchess of Devonshire. The Manners couple had the reputation of being the most handsome pair in all of Ireland.

[96]   Rotunda Hospital, the oldest maternity hospital in the British Isles, founded in 1745 by Bartholomew Mosse and housed from 1757 in a new building (known as the 'Rotunda'). In the 1780s, a set of assembly-rooms were established for public functions such as balls and concerts, proceeds from which went to fund the hospital.

to unite beneficence with so many amiable qualities. Her Grace sent me the next day, by her first gentleman-usher, a purse of thirty guineas.

The Duke of Leinster[97] was not less generous on this occasion; he brought me himself twenty guineas. His greatness of soul, his bounty, are written with indelible characters in the hearts of many unhappy creatures, whom he relieves during the severity of the winter, both in town and at his country-seats, in a manner as judicious as charitable. I myself saw one day an act of humanity, which has inspired me with the most profound veneration for that nobleman. As he passed on horseback through Dame-street, an unlucky servant, whose foot had slipt as he was getting behind a coach, fell between the hind-wheel and the body. Happily for the man, the Duke at that instant was by the coach; he alights, and flying on the horses, stops them, and takes out the poor fellow, whom one turn more of the wheel would have crushed to death. Such an action is above praise: how excellent in itself, but how sublime in a great Lord, and how proud must I be, to have met with such protectors!

I should not have staid so long in Ireland, had it not been for the illness of my wife who was pregnant; but having followed the advice given me to go to Newry and Drogheda, a trip which did not defray the expenses, she fell so dangerously ill in this last town, that her surgeon Mr. Roger, thinking her child dead, decided it was necessary to deliver her by force. He had already got his instruments ready; when, fortunately, after some symptoms, he waited two days more before he came to so painful an operation; and having employed that interval in stupes and fomentations, he at last became assured that the child was alive. This unexpected turn calmed my uneasiness, and comforted me on the fate of a wife to whom I am bound by so many ties. I am under the greatest obligations to this skilful and prudent gentleman, whom I could never prevail upon to accept of any fee; and this opportunity is the only one I have in my power to convince him of my gratitude.

It was not only this illness, but a very disagreeable accident that still retarded my journey. I had been advised to send my wife and daughter to bathe in the sea; and they were consequently gone to a small house I had hired for them on the sea-coast, two miles from Dublin. They had with them a servant called Francis Lombardi, a native of London, the son of a late dentist of that name, and

---

[97]   William Robert Fitzgerald, Duke of Leinster (1749–1804).

whose mother then lived in Dublin. One day this fellow disappeared, carrying away with him some of our goods, worth upwards of sixty guineas; and among other things, a ring-watch surrounded with diamonds. I advertised the theft in the news-papers, offering two guineas reward to such as could supply me with sufficient information, that I might recover my effects. Four months after I received a letter, when I was at Liverpool, acquainting me that a Mr. Crosthwaite, watch-maker, Grafton street, Dublin,[98] had in his possession the said watch, which he had stopped from a lawyer, who said he had bought it for four guineas of a vagabond at Belfast. I immediately wrote to claim it; and offered to return the four guineas, besides the two guineas reward; but all my endeavours have proved ineffectual. In vain did I make application to all the persons with whom I had the honour to be acquainted; in vain did I write a second letter last year to Mr. David de la Touche,[99] who, undoubtedly, has not received my letter, or else he would have favoured me with an answer. Unless some worthy persons, feeling a proper indignation at seeing a foreigner so ill treated, will be so kind as to interpose in this matter, if it be in their power, I must give up the hope of ever possessing again an object which I valued, not so much for the worth of it, as for remembrances dear to me.

Having been retarded more than four months by all these untoward circumstances, I at length set out, and rapidly travelling through Liverpool, Manchester and Birmingham, repaired to Oxford, where I made a considerable stay.

One day a gentleman came and desired me to go and spend the evening at about eight or nine miles distance. He would not tell the place, but assured me that a carriage would take me thither, and I should not repent my visit. In effect, how great was my surprise and admiration, when I found myself conveyed to the magnificent palace of Blenheim, where Their graces the Duke and Duchess of Marlborough[100] welcomed me in the most affable manner. The Duchess herself vouchsafed to shew me the apartments, and point out all curious pieces they

---

[98]   A watchmaker John Crosthwaite had his shop at 27 Grafton Street in 1783.

[99]   David La Touche – this was the name and surname of successive representatives of a dynasty of Dublin bankers descended from Huguenot emigrants. Boruwłaski probably wrote his letter to David the third (–1817), a member of the Irish Parliament.

[100]   George Spencer, Duke of Marlborough (1739–1817). His wife was Caroline Russell (1743–1811), daughter of John, Duke of Bedford.

contain. I played on the guitar; and, when I took my leave, the Duke ordered his chaplain to present me with a very pretty steel chain, and a bank-note of ten pounds.

At length I returned to London in March 1786, after about three years absence. I met there with the Grand General of Lithuania, the Count Ogiński, who had shewn me so much kindness during my stay at Paris. He seemed to take much pleasure in seeing me again, and promised to assist me on all occasions with his name and credit.

This was a most favourable opportunity for me to perform another concert, under inspection of this nobleman, so approved for talents of every kind, who had designed to teach me the first element of music. The day appointed was the 30th June. His Royal Highness the Prince of Wales promised to be present. He had at dinner with him, on that day, His Highness the Prince de Mecklenbourg,[101] and wishing to shew me to this Prince, he sent his carriage for me. I found Their Highnesses at table, with whom I sat down a full hour, and should have staid much longer, if the fear of wearing out the patience of the public, who expected me to the concert, had not obliged me to retire. When I took my leave, His Royal Highness was so kind as to reiterate his promise of coming; but something unforeseen hindered him, and I was deprived of that honour.

Though this concert was tolerably well performed, and before a chosen assembly yet I should have suffered a loss, if the generous Count Ogiński had not paid Mr. Gallini all the charges of it.

About that time I was informed that His Grace the Duke of Marlborough wished to have one of my shoes, and place it in his cabinet among other rarities. I had too much reason to be flattered with this nobleman's affability not to send him a pair of them immediately, to which I joined the only pair of boots I had made for me, which I had brought from Poland. His Grace was so well pleased with this mark of attention, that the next day he sent me a bank-note of 20 l.[102]

It was then in agitation to give the public an history of my life. Many persons of quality, as well as naturalists, pressed me to undertake it; and I received a number of subscriptions, as soon as my project was known; even His Royal Highness

---

[101]   Adolphus Frederick IV, Prince of Mecklenburg-Strelitz (1738–1794), the brother of Queen Charlotte and the uncle of the future George IV.

[102]   Pounds.

the Prince of Wales was graciously pleased to be at the head of the subscribers. Therefore I ought only to mind this task, and do my best endeavours to render such work, according to the very small abilities I had, worthy the patronage of so many illustrious persons, who condescended to interest themselves for me. But let me be permitted to pass over in silence all the difficulties and crosses I met with, in an undertaking which required many recollections, and more time than was imagined at first. I will only say, and that with the utmost gratitude, that I could never have brought it about, without the bounty of the Princess Lubomirska,[103] who deigned to enter into the minutest detail of my situation, and on seeing I was exposed to vexations from ill-natured creditors ready to prosecute me, asked for an account of my debts, which, though they amounted to upwards of fifty guineas, she was so kind as to discharge for me. I can never forget such an act of beneficence, since, by restoring me to tranquillity, it has put it in my power to finish this performance.

I am come at last to a conclusion of the principal events of my life. I have described, as much as in my power, my adventures, my sentiments, the unfolding of my intellectual faculties, have gone back to the time of each event. On examining my heart, I have still found in it the same sentiments, the same source from whence arose my pleasures, my errors and misfortunes, and following this current, have discovered a very comfortable truth: that a man of feeling never regrets those actions which originate from tenderness of sentiment, when unaccompanied by self-reproach. If a look on my children affect me; if a glance of a dear wife, who has been so long my adored companion, and is now become a sincere friend, recall to my mind a sweet remembrance, I feel a starting tear, which would be the tear of happiness, did not other intrusive fears disturb these delightful moments.

After having spoken of what I have done and thought, may I be permitted to fix my reader's attention for a moment upon my present situation, to open my heart before my benefactors, and so many persons who take interest in me, to disclose its inquietudes, agitations and fears? May I hope, without being accused

---

[103] Isabella (Elżbieta) Lubomirska née Czartoryska (1736–1816) – the daughter of Augustus, one of the most powerful individuals of the Polish-Lithuanian Commonwealth, the wife of Stanisław, Grand Marshal of the Crown, a relative and friend (later enemy) of Stanisław Augustus, and one of the most celebrated Polish ladies of the eighteenth century. She was in London starting in May 1787.

of presumption, that a noble and generous nation, in the midst of which I have, for these six years, found an agreeable retreat, enjoyed a multiplicity of resources, and a peaceful existence, will deign to compassionate the fate of a being, stamped by nature herself on the coin of the marvellous, and whose life presents a texture of events, almost all of which have flowed from an excess of sensibility?

I have spent my youth in pleasures and opulence. At this epoch, when nature claims her rights, reflection and good advice have had the power to draw me from a licentious life, and teach me how to surmount the vague desires which tormented me; but neither reason nor obstacles were able to free me from love, when a truly deserving person was the object of my passion. I forgot in one moment what I owed to my benefactress, to myself, to consistency; it seemed that love would not admit any other sentiment in my heart; I became ungrateful; I left without regret a house, which, some time before, I could not have given up but on feeling a mortal grief; at last, I united myself to her for whom I had sacrificed all, and I was at the height of my wishes. His Majesty the King of Poland, vouchsafed to favour me with one hundred and twenty ducats annuity. On finding this to be insufficient, my friends prevailed on me to travel; I have been everywhere kindly received, and agreeably entertained, everywhere loaded with presents; but all is swallowed up by considerable expenses which a long residence in towns required.

At length, I arrived in England. How shall I express the sentiments of gratitude, deeply impressed in my heart? Here I excite a kind of enthusiasms; a calculation is immediately formed on the generosity of some particular benefactors, without considering the enormous expenses unavoidable in that sort of life I was obliged to lead. It is reported that I have laid out six thousands pounds in the funds; this report reaches my own country, it gets ground there; hence it is concluded, I want the King's favours no longer, and my annuity is cut off; in that very moment, when Lady Egremont deigns openly to protect a subscription, with a view to procure me a subsistence, when the Princess Lubomirska, affected at my distress, clears my debts, when, perhaps, I am upon the verge of being for ever deprived of the friendship and counsels of a generous man,[104] who, through regard for distinguished persons my protectors in Poland,

---

[104]   This is quite a mysterious sentence. If we are to believe what is reported by Catherine Hutton, as confirmed in a letter from Boruwłaski to Bukaty, the only person accompanying

has been so kind as to accompany me in my travels, and has reaped no other benefit for all his troubles, but to see himself accused of being prejudicial to my welfare; whereas it is but too true, that if I had duly attended to his counsels, if yielding to his remonstrances, I had not so often trusted to people who abused my credulous disposition, I should at least have had some resources.

Such is the picture of what is past: it is easy to see how pains are mingled with pleasures, fears with hopes. But what is the fate I am to expect? Am I doomed to be for ever the sport of necessity, the slave of the moment? What do I say? Though I should submit to this humiliating idea, would it lead to the hope of securing, in future, a decent maintenance for my wife and children? I have but a weak constitution, the weight of years grows every day more pressing; should I be snatched away from my family, what will become of them? Whose assistance can they claim? Am I destined to have, on my last day, nothing in view, but the misery and woe of all that is dear to me? These are the pains and inquietudes which assail my heart, and dash with bitterness the moments of joy that I derive from my family. Had I been formed like other mortals, I could, like most of them, have subsisted by industry and labour; but my stature has irrevocably excluded me from the common circle of society. Nay, but few people only seem to take notice of my being a man, an honest man, a man of feeling. How painful are these reflections!

O beneficent and generous nation! Should I sink under my griefs I recommend to you my wife and children, my children, who came into life among you; whose glory it is to be your countrymen, if I am not at the end of my career, then I must repair to other climates, where yielding to my destiny, I will submit to that fate which seems to await me; but I will take with me everywhere, will cherish, and carefully keep in the inmost recesses of my heart, the grateful sentiments which your repeated favours have excited in me.

FINIS

***

Boruwłaski in his travels was Mr de Trouville, conjectured to be Isalina's uncle, and so he would be the individual referred to here.

Report Delivered to the French Royal Academy of Sciences by the Count de Tressan, Paris 1760

Translated from French by A. Grześkowiak-Krwawicz, D. Sax

M. Borwslasky,[105] a Polish nobleman, arrived in Lunéville in the entourage of the Countess Humiecka, widow of the Grand Sword-Bearer of the Polish Crown, a relative of His Majesty the King of Poland. This young gentleman can be seen as the most curious being that has ever existed in nature; Bébé the Polish King's dwarf no longer has any trait that may be found surprising once one has gotten to know him.

Mr. Borwslasky is 22 years of age and but 28 inches high – at this height he is built impeccably, nature has not forgotten about anything, and he is not deformed by any misshapen body part. His head is well-proportioned, his eyes beautiful and full of fire, all of his traits are agreeable, his physiognomy mild and bright, indicating gaiety, politeness, and all the finesse of his spirit. His figure is straight and shapely, his knees, legs, and feet have the right proportions for a well-built and strong man. I know from individuals who served him that he is of full virility. He can easily raise with one hand weights that seem significant compared to his stature. He enjoys perfect health, drinks only water, eats little, sleeps well, and is resistant to fatigue. He dances aptly, is adroit and light; nature has not refused anything to this graceful Creature; it even seems that it sought to make amends for his extremely small height with the graces embellishing his entire personality, including ones continually discovered in his intellect.

He joins in the most graceful manner in subtle and spirited repartees, he speaks highly sensibly of what he has seen, and he has a very good memory; his judgement is sound, his heart sensitive, capable of gratitude and attachment; he does not show rage or malice. He is extremely complacent and greatly values politeness shown to him, especially when he is talked to as a 22-year-old man and with the decorum due to a nobleman. But he does not show impatience or moodiness to those who, somewhat taking advantage of his small size, permit themselves to joke or talk to him as with a child.

---

[105] de Tressan distorts Boruwłaski's true name considerably, consistently writing 'Borwslasky.'

The father and mother of M. Borwslasky are considerably above average height. They have six children, the eldest of whom is but thirty-four inches high, the second, Joseph (whom my report pertains to), is but 28 inches high, the three younger brothers who came into the world one year after the next are all around 5 feet 6 inches high, strong and well-shaped. The sixth child is a girl, nearly six years old, said to be of charming figure and face, only 20 or 21 inches high. She moves and talks as freely as other children of her age and promises to be just as sharp as her second brother.

It is worth knowing that the father and mother of these children looked upon the two oldest like unfortunate whims of nature and left them without education. Only starting about two years ago did the Countess Humiecka and another lady relation of hers take the two young men under their protection. I do not know the condition of the elder, but I could not look upon the one I am reporting about without admiration that he was able to attain such knowledge in the short span of two years. He is very well educated on issues of the Catholic religion he professes, reads and writes well, knows arithmetic, and even has a sense of order that allows him to maintain in the best condition accounts of everything he has and spends. He is extremely adept at all he undertakes to do, and one can easily notice that he never compromises himself by undertaking what is beyond his strength. In four months he learned German sufficiently for his needs and French quite thoroughly, to express himself with ease and in sophisticated phrases. In a word, there is nothing childish about him, nor any of the weaknesses and mental infirmity which the King of Poland's dwarf manifests so often, more often than a 4-year-old child.

Here we should stress a few more significant differences between the two dwarfs. The one belonging to the King of Poland was born of a farmer woman from the Mountains of Vosges in the seventh month of pregnancy. As an infant he was not even 8 inches tall; a sabot half-full of wool served as his cradle for more than a year. Bébé is 20 years old and would have received the best education had he been able to gain from it. He is currently 36 inches tall, his back seems to be bent with age, his skin is wrinkled, one shoulder blade sticks out much further than the other, his aquiline nose became monstrous, his congenital apophysis[106] has developed all the way into the deformation of the upper part of his body; his

---

[106] bony protrusions.

intellect is by no means well developed, he has never successfully had the ideas of religion instilled in him, or taught to recognize letters, he had never managed to perform the slightest work; he is stupid, irascible, and Descartes' system concerning the soul of animals would be easier to prove by citing the existence of Bébé than the existence of the monkey or poodle. What I have reported here about M. Borwslasky, on the contrary, shows the young Pole to have a mild and very intelligent mind. I will even admit that I have always observed Bébé with the repugnance and concealed horror usually inspired by the degradation of our existence, while the young Pole, in contrast, instils pleasure with his appearance and intellect, he arouses interest in his feelings, and finally evokes just tenderness and a desire to soothe all pain and indignity such as his fate may entail.

***

And here are the highly extraordinary circumstances of the births of the three Polish children. The Countess Humiecka and many individuals from her entourage have assured me of them. I, in turn, deemed them too interesting to refuse myself the honour of giving an account of them to the Academy. Madame Borwslaska, the mother, gave birth to all six of her children at the proper time. The three boys who are today of tall stature were born at the normal size of 18 to 22 inches, and all the parts of their body were well-shaped, free and fully developed. When the three dwarfs were born, the children were barely of human shape when coming into the world – the head, hidden between the shoulders so that the tip was on their level, gave the upper part of their body the shape of a square; the thighs and shins, crossed and pressed to the tailbone and to the mons pubis, made the lower part oval. Everything together represented a shapeless mass as long as it was wide, which had nothing human about it but for the features of the face. These three children developed gradually, but none of them remained deformed, on the contrary they are ideally proportional and well built, never wore corsets, and no trick was used to improve nature. These reports do not suggest that deformations in the shape of the womb may have harmed the foetus and hampered its development, because after giving birth to two dwarfs the mother bore three large and properly developed boys, and after them a girl quite similar to the first two, who came into the world in the same shape as they.

The Countess Humiecka should soon come to Paris, where she is travelling to seek assistance for pains in the right knee. After arriving she will presumably consult M. Morand, and she honoured me with a promise to bring M. Borwslasky to the Academy, for him to be examined there. I admit that I am so greatly moved by the fate of this young nobleman that I felt it was my duty to have the honour of reporting his person to the Assembly. Your love for humanity, the consideration you have for foreigners, will make this examination more satisfactory than disagreeable for this young man, made so interesting by his mature mind and mild and good manners.

I insistently urged the Countess Humiecka to try to supply detailed information to the Academy about the status of Madame Borwslaska during her pregnancies and the account of the accoucheuse or midwife who received the births. M. Morand[107] may reiterate that insistence in order to receive new reports that may perhaps contribute to formulating some sort of conjecture about the causes of the phenomenon.

Lunéville, 3 December 1759

---

[107] Sauveur-François Morand (1697–1773), French surgeon, member of the French Academy of Sciences.

Index

Printed and bound by CPI Group (UK) Ltd, Croydon, CR0 4YY

18/10/2024

01776271-0001